P9-BYV-243

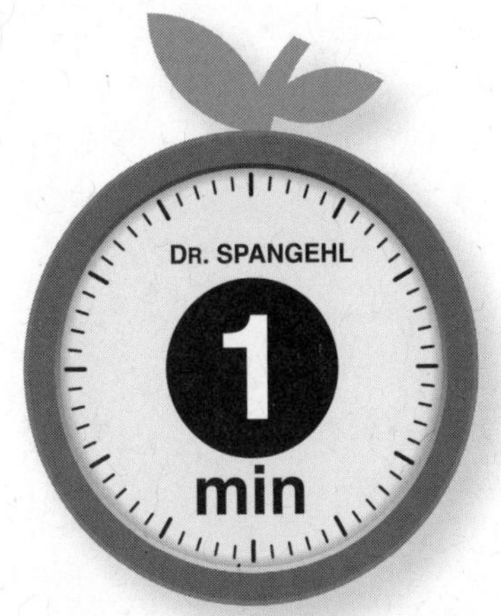


# one minute medicine

YOUR EFFORTLESS GUIDE TO VIBRANT HEALTH

WERNER SPANGEHL, M.D.

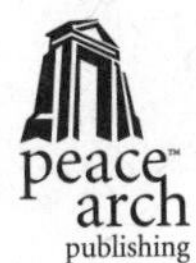

978-0-9869430-1-0



The author is grateful to Jim Murphy, David Bentall, Dave Phillips, Dr. Davidicus Wong and Jay Carty for permission to quote their works. (See Reference section)



Printed on Forestry Stewardship Council (FSC) ancient forest friendly paper which is produced acid free and chlorine free with 100% recycled fibers

Printed in Canada

## Dedication

*This book is dedicated to my enthusiastic and inspirational children: **Tori**, **Madeline**, and **Peter**. Their future is bright, and it is my hope and prayer that they reach their potential to make the world a better place.*

*I also dedicate this work to their mother—my beloved wife, **Vivian**, who has blessed my life for over thirty years and enables me to strive for Magna Vita!*

# PRAISE FOR ONE MINUTE MEDICINE

"ONE MINUTE MEDICINE is an engaging, authoritative guide for anyone seeking to live a healthier, more fulfilling life. Dr. Werner Spangehl offers expert, down-to-earth advice on every major aspect of health -- body, mind, spirit. I advise you to buy two copies -- one for you, and one for your doctor."
— **Larry Dossey**, MD, Physician, Speaker and Author: *HEALING WORDS and THE POWER OF PREMONITIONS*

Dr. Spangehl is leading people to healthy lifestyles, which is what we all need!!
— **Joe Sakic**, Former Captain Colorado Avalanche and Canadian Men's Olympic Hockey Team

This is such valuable information when it comes to understanding how we can play a key role in our own health and wellness. It is important to implement preventive measures in our daily lives to ensure optimum health and longevity.
— **Dianne L. Watts**, Mayor, City of Surrey, British Columbia

Werner has written a practical, inspiring handbook for healthy living. As his water ski training partner for nearly a decade, I can heartily endorse him as a Doc who lives what he prescribes!
— **David C Bentall**, Author, Speaker, Family Business Advisor and Life Coach.

This stuff really works! ONE MINUTE MEDICINE is advice about simple choices for health and happiness from a man that I trust. In fact I'd say this is the way he lives his life. Werner has made the keys to great health and peak performance easy to understand. I hope all of my friends and clients will have a chance to read One Minute Medicine because if they follow his advice it WILL make their lives better!

"The things that are easy to do are also easy not to do."— Author unknown

— **Dave Phillips**, Author, executive mentor and speaker
Former member and coach of Canada's National Freestyle Ski team, and Guinness World record holder

Dr. Spangehl's book ONE MINUTE MEDICINE is a simple yet powerful guide that examines many of the recognized as well as unrecognized factors that affect optimal health. This is a vibrant book that can transform your life from a doc who walks the talk!

— **Jim Murphy**, Author, Inner Excellence (McGraw-Hill),
Mental Skills Coach to PGA and LPGA Tour players

Having endured my fair share of health issues over the years; including a mild stroke, I have pledged to take better care of myself in recent years! Recently I read the book ONE MINUTE MEDICINE and I was pleasantly surprised at how Doctor Spangehl was able to deliver an engaging story to his audience while providing readers with concrete and achievable guidance for a healthier more enjoyable life.

— **Tom Watson**, Businessman, International Speaker, Best Selling Author of *MAN SHOES*

As a Catholic priest, I often speak of the human body as being a temple of the Holy Spirit. Dr Spangehl's book has given me layer upon layer of practical appreciation of the reverence, respect and responsibility due the human body as such a temple.
— **Fr. Stanley Galvon**, Pastor, Star of the Sea Catholic Parish, South Surrey/ White Rock, British Columbia

Fitness is my business and my passion. And over the years, Dr. Werner Spangehl has been a trusted source of health information for my family and me. I feel that his book, ONE MINUTE MEDICINE will be helpful to anyone looking to improve their overall health and fitness.
— **James Newman**, Founder and CEO, Fitness Town—Your Fitness Equipment Experts

ONE MINUTE MEDICINE is a remarkable consolidation of information that is current and state of the art. It will be a great asset to recommend to patients, when they are confused about what the media hits them with. It really is pretty simple and I love the "one-minute" approach. Baby steps to healthy habits. I think it is a great reference for docs too, as we are role models for our patients, families, children, and each other.
— **Dr. Connie Ruffo**, Family Physician and Founder of "Physicians Advocating Wellness", White Rock, BC
Former Director, "Physician Health Program", British Columbia

"A great book from a doc who walks the talk! Through the voice of David, I was reminded that what makes us happy and healthy are very similar, inter-related and simple. A must read that is both universally appealing and unique."
— **Jackie Smith**, Executive Director, Peace Arch Hospital and Community Health Foundation

When my mother's doctor retired, I requested a referral to a real doctor—one who still believed in and practiced the original Hippocratic Oath of "firstly, do no harm". One who had a great bedside manner, kept updating his knowledge base, and was open to the benefits of good nutrition, exercise, and other such complementary modalities.

What I really had in mind, I guess, was someone like my dear, departed father—a true family doctor—who, in the 1930's, had been educated at the prestigious German universities of Munich and Freiburg.

It turned out that the retired doctor steered us right, because we totally lucked out in Dr. Spangehl. Despite being deceptively young looking when we first met, it was clear that he was knowledgeable, caring and totally focused on his patients.

When he comes through that door at the office, it is like he is delighted to see an old friend after a long absence. At the end of the visit, he gently gives us a short synopsis about how to improve on some of our life-choices in regards to our diet, exercise, stress-reducing methods, blood-pressure and cholesterol levels, or whatever applies to the individual.

I found his book to be as readily accessible as he is. ONE MINUTE MEDICINE is so readable and informative in outlining the determinants of physical, mental and emotional health that you could easily finish it in one go, like a good thriller. The book will help you to find balance, harmony and optimal health as you age.

There are the *12 Habits of Healthy People* that go down well, without preaching as well as the attention-grabbing one minute message boxes that remind us of what is really important. The story of David's heart attack serves as an analogy of what can easily happen to any of us. Since not

everyone can be Dr. Spangehl's patient, ONE MINUTE MEDICINE will allow you to benefit from his wisdom in your own home.
— **Kareen Zebroff**; Yogini Emeritus (Television host of Kareen's Yoga, 1970-1986 ); Best-selling Author of 10 books in 14 languages on Yoga and Nutrition; Teacher/Practitioner of GNM (German New Medicine).

This engaging book is a labour of love for GP, Werner Spangehl. There are two side by side narratives. In one he tells the compelling story of how one man and his family deals with his premature heart attack at the age of 42. Embedded in this story is a book called "12 Habits of Healthy People" that synthesizes the latest research on every aspect of health optimization. This book within a book outlines small practical steps to upgrade your health and at the same time summarizes the latest research to support the health benefits of those steps. For example, there are "Incidental" and "Better than Nothing" Exercises. There are also realistic down to earth guides to nutrition, meditation, sleep hygiene, spiritual awareness, work enjoyment, life-long learning and much more. Step by step Werner is showing his patients how to make the long term changes that will result in a much happier and healthier life. Werner is not interested in the quick fix but in the slow permanent lifestyle changes that will prevent serious illness and ensure a much higher quality of life.
— **Carolyn DeMarco**, MD, author and GP

*Praise for ONE MINUTE MEDICINE continued on page 343.*

# TABLE OF CONTENTS

# FOREWORD

Dr Werner Spangehl's compassionate approach and consummate professionalism are evident on every page of this book. His narrative is readable, informative and engaging and it is based on both sound research and real life experience. His characters live the lives and face the challenges that we all face. They are our friends and our neighbours - they are us.

One Minute Medicine uses one minute messages for us to focus on for as much or as little time as we may have available. Werner is able to weave the many strands of complementary and traditional practices into an understandable fabric that we can all identify with and find comfort in. It addresses our vulnerabilities, and shows a path towards balance and an integrated holistic sense of self, and at the same time it addresses our global challenges of personal and planetary sustainability. He shows us that little changes can make a big difference. Incrementalism works—small changes made today will have a profound impact on tomorrow. They are the foundations of change in our lifestyles. One Minute Medicine reaffirms the power which we have to effect positive change in our lives, in our families and in our communities. It is both reassuring and empowering.

For many of us, from the moment the alarm clock calls until we close our eyes, our day to day world seems to become ever more complex and demanding. Often the last person we take care of is ourselves and that can mean that we sacrifice our personal health and well-being. As a husband, father, former foster parent, probation officer, Mayor, Member of the Legislative Assembly, and as a Cabinet Minister, I have experienced the demands that often consume our well-being.

I have known Dr. Werner Spangehl for over two decades and I have appreciated and admired his ability to express the critical needs of day to day health care in a personal and understandable fashion. He uses his knowledge to partner with patients and communities to develop understandable workable strategies that lead to healthier lives and healthier communities. One Minute Medicine is an inspiring, easy to read book that is both optimistic and encouraging.

Dr. Spangehl is a leader in the Peace Arch community and through One Minute Medicine shares his knowledge and enthusiasm for an active and healthy way of life with all of us.

**Gordon Hogg**, BA, MEd, PhD (candidate)

As the minister of Health Promotion in B.C. (ActNow BC) (2005-07) Gordon led an integrated collaborative approach to community health that received acclaim from the World Health Organization, the Public Health Association of Canada, the Health Council of Canada and the Dieticians of Canada. He is the son of one of the pioneer family doctors in South Surrey—White Rock and his first lessons in community and medicine came from accompanying his father on house calls.

# ACKNOWLEDGMENTS

I would like to thank my editorial review panel who took the time to give me honest and useful feedback on the draft manuscript that resulted in countless improvements to the story, the layout, and the readability of this work. This group includes Ken Bray, Kathie Spangehl, Kathy Kinloch, Harvey Strecker, Henri Lorieau, Ryan Payne, Brenda Hefford, Steve Larigakis, Connie Ruffo, Lourens Perold, Petr Polasek, Sean Rose, Donna Herringer, Tim Barker, and my Brothers in Slalom, especially David Bentall and Dave Phillips.

I am very grateful to my parents, Erhardt and Karin Spangehl, as well as my siblings, Marita Bray and Mark Spangehl for their support and encouragement.

I would also like to acknowledge Vivian Spangehl for her ability to make healthy foods taste great and for all the nutritious meals she makes for our family and friends. She provided the recipes in this book for fabulous Flax Snax, potent Power Pucks and Vivacious Vivian's Vitality Muffins!

Special thanks to Jennifer Boyle, yogini extraordinaire, and Founder of Bikram Yoga, White Rock, for scheduling the time for numerous photo shoots—each with more incredible poses than the time before.

I am grateful to Adrienne Thiessen of Gemini Visuals Creative Photography for her expertise in taking the yoga images as well as the shots for the book jacket and website.

Ken Bray is a Canadian Landscape painter who provided several of the non-yoga images and rendered all of the images on Photoshop. (www.kenbray.ca)

Margaret Davidson is an experienced story editor based in Vancouver who helped me to shape the original manuscript into a more succinct book. I would like to thank her for her patience in going back and forth over the manuscript until we felt it contained enough material to inspire and inform and not too much to overwhelm or dilute the central message.

Katharine Herringer and Iván Álvarez de Lorenzana of Multibird Branding are based in Majorca, Spain. I appreciated all the Skype meetings and e-mails as well as their creative enthusiasm on the design and layout of the One Minute Medicine book and Website.

I would like to thank Phil Whitmarsh and Carolyn Madison at Self Publishing, Inc.—a division of RJ Communications in New York, and Jorge Rocha, Curwin Friesen and others at Friesens in Canada for their assistance in the publishing and printing of this book.

I am also thankful to Dr. Terry Anderson, who has given me helpful advice and leads on the writing, editing, publishing, and marketing of this work from its very inception in 2001.

Every community has its local heroes—ordinary people who give of themselves for the benefit of others. Most of these extraordinary people are unrecognized. As this book celebrates ordinary people achieving *Magna Vita* I would like to recognize some of these people in my community. This includes families who provide foster care or adopt children who otherwise would not reach their potential, single mothers of kids with special needs, volunteers in food banks and soup kitchens, coaches and managers of various sports teams that freely offer their time and talent, a colleague who regularly does medical mission work in Africa, and the conductor of our church choir, to name but a few.

I would also like to acknowledge my office staff who organize my workdays: Sheila, Phyllis, Ashley, Amanda, Alex and Emily.

Finally, I could not have written this book without the input from all of my patients who have moved me and inspired me over the years; it has been a privilege for me to share your journeys, your joys, and your sorrows. Collectively, you have taught me valuable lessons about courage, determination, patience, joy, triumph, resilience, and acceptance. My hope is that our interactions have equally been of service to you and that the lessons reflected in this book will also be helpful to others.

# INTRODUCTION

This book is intended to give *useful information about a healthy lifestyle* to anyone who may need it. Being fit and vital has been shown to dramatically improve general health, mitigate chronic health conditions, and increase life expectancy. The benefits of a healthy lifestyle include a reduced need for prescription medications, fewer hospitalizations, and greatly improved energy, happiness, and functional capability at any age.

*One Minute Medicine* is the story of David Mackenzie and his journey of recovery from a heart attack. There are many vignettes and anecdotes in these pages that are drawn from real life events. However, this is a work of fiction and any names or specific examples that may resemble actual people or events are purely coincidental. Most are composites drawing on several cases that are pulled together to illustrate a particular point.

One Minute Medicine also contains excerpts of an instructional booklet entitled *12 Habits of Healthy People*. This is intended as reference material on factors such as diet, exercise, and sleep that broadly influence health. Its sections can be read in the sequence that they are printed, or they can be looked up as needed at a later date. Pages can be dog eared and passages can be pondered.

Throughout the book, "One Minute Messages" can be found. These are summaries that include practical suggestions on how to achieve goals.

**One minute message**

When skimming through the book, the reader can pick out these "One Minute Messages" and later return to the rest of the information on that habit. The book is designed both for readers who have specific goals such as improved diet, fitness, sleep, weight loss, or smoking cessation, as well as readers looking for an overall guide to achieving good health and longevity.

While as inclusive as possible regarding the determinants of health, this book is designed to be *concise rather than comprehensive and accessible without being unduly technical.* There is information in these pages that will benefit every reader, yet each of the topics can be explored much further. Think of it as a starting point to better health. If something piques your curiosity, there are references listed for additional information.

Our attitudes and beliefs play important roles in healing and wellness. These aspects are explored in the fascinating fields of mind-body medicine, placebo literature, the biology of gene expression, and psychoneuroimmunology (the study of interactions between the mind and the nervous and immune systems). In other words, there are solid scientific explanations as to how people can feel more vigorous, strengthen their immune systems to fight infections and disease, and even slow the aging process by following the habits of healthy living. Some of this biology will be summarized to better understand these conclusions.

There are also a number of recipes, a "diet" to follow, and exercises that can be tried. There will be opportunities for readers to share their stories and recipes on the website: www.oneminutemedicine.com.

The take-home message from this book is a simple one. A series of steps will enable you to make a profound difference in your health, allowing you to lead a full and vital life, whatever your age.

Moreover, the return on investment is high. Surprisingly, the positive choices that we make every day are often enjoyable and not particularly difficult. They can decrease our risk of disease as well as improve recovery when illness occurs. In addition, following *12 Habits* can actually slow the aging process, specifically deteriorating conditions such as *musculoskeletal disease* (arthritis, weakness, osteoporosis, and poor balance, resulting in falls and fractures); *neurodegenerative diseases* (dementia and Parkinson's disease); *cardiovascular disease* (stroke and heart attacks) and *cancer*. At the same time, our new choices provide us health benefits that are multiple and varied as there is an elegant consistency in the recommendations. This book provides a framework for how to live our lives to the optimum.

The purpose of this book is to outline the pitfalls contributing to ill health, suggest alternatives that can lead to better health, and offer you the means to make positive changes in your own life. I encourage you to reflect on David's journey, as my hope is that this book will motivate and inspire every reader to further improve his or her health and wellbeing.

# CHAPTER 1

*"Health is the greatest wealth."*

**Ralph Waldo Emerson**
(1803–1882), American poet, philosopher, lecturer, and essayist

"What have you got?" asked Dr. Harper. An ambulance crew had just burst through the doors of the emergency room wheeling a man on a stretcher.

"Forty-two-year-old Caucasian male, found in V-tach after his car crashed into a mountainside this side of Squamish. We defibrillated at 200 joules and started the amiodarone protocol. BP 100 over 60, pulse 110, O2 sats 96 percent on 5 liters by mask," replied the paramedic crisply.

"Good. Stat ECG, CBC, lytes, urea, creatinine, LFTs, troponin, and cardiac enzymes," Harper barked to the nurse routinely, as though she were giving a shopping list to her husband.

Immobilized on the stretcher, cold and profoundly scared, was David Mackenzie, whose brown eyes darted nervously around the ER and then fixed upon Harper like someone clinging to a capsized life-raft in a violent sea. "I'm Doctor Harper," the emergency room physician said to David reassuringly. "It looks as if you may have had a heart attack, but we're going to take very good care of you."

Jillian Harper understood the fear that her patients faced. Over the last sixteen years she had seen thousands of patients with all kinds of complaints arrive through those ER doors; some were people she knew, and several did not survive their illnesses and injuries. All too often, she had witnessed the emotional vulnerability of patients with a life threatening condition having to come face to face with their own mortality.

David spent the next few days in a surreal blur. He was aware of what was happening, but it had not sunk in; he could not accept that he had had a heart attack. *Man, I could have died!* he kept thinking. *I could still die.*

David thought back to early Monday morning when he had taken the Sea to Sky Highway from Whistler to Vancouver. He'd been driving too fast; David had recently been made a partner at the law firm Kane Wallace & Sullivan and was late for a meeting. He had been smoking a cigarette and feeling that the smoke was burning his throat. He could not take a deep breath, as his chest felt tight and would not expand. Suddenly drenched in a cold sweat, David became aware of his heart pounding painfully in his chest, pushing up to his throat. The tightness did not relent even after he had ripped off his tie. The pressure then moved up into his ears and he felt sure his head was going to burst. He remembered thinking he was going to die as his vision blurred and he felt his car go off the road. Thoughts ceased as his world went black.

As David lay in his hospital bed, an expression his German-speaking mother often used came back to him. "Glűck im Unglűck," she would say. "You have good fortune in your misfortune."

He now realized how true that had been on the day of his heart attack. A police cruiser planning to pull him over for speeding had recognized that he was in trouble and had radioed for an ambulance. David might well have died had the ambulance with Advanced Life Support not arrived within a few minutes. The paramedics immediately recognized his dangerous heart irregularity and were able to correct his heart beat with their defibrillator. They started an IV, gave him appropriate medications and an oxygen mask and transported him to St. Luke's Hospital and Health Sciences Centre in North Vancouver.

St. Luke's was the major referral hospital for the area and

had an excellent cardiac program. Because David was young and previously well he was treated with primary angioplasty. The procedure was straightforward. A catheter was inserted through the radial artery of his right wrist and advanced to the heart, where dye was injected into the coronary arteries; these are the small but tremendously important arteries that supply the heart itself with blood and oxygen. This study demonstrated that David had a significant blockage in one artery, and Dr. Schreiber, his cardiologist, was able to open the blockage with a balloon catheter and then deploy a wire mesh stent into the narrowed area to keep the artery open.

.........................................................................

David Mackenzie awoke to a soft and steady beeping sound that marched in exact time with his heart rate. The smell of clean hospital linen and the sterile odour of disinfectants filled his nostrils. He opened his eyes slowly and began taking in the clinical surroundings of the Intensive Care Unit of St. Luke's Hospital. He had tubes and wires connecting him to medical equipment and could see a TV monitor above his bed with multi-coloured lines and blips moving from left to right across the screen. His eyes drifted around the room. Although he was in a three-sided ICU bay, he could see a few other patients lying in similar circumstances, some of whom were attached to breathing machines.

David tried to call to the nurse nearby but his lips and mouth were parched, and his voice cracked. She soon looked up and motioned that she had heard him and would be right over. As she made her way towards his bed, David noticed that all the other patients were gray-haired. Old. "What am I doing here?" he asked himself.

The nurse had reached his bed. Her nametag identified her as *Mary Ann*, and her eyes were warm and compassionate. "So you've decided to re-join the living, have you, Mr. Mackenzie? You suffered a heart attack while you were driving. Your car might not make it, but the doctors think you will!"

She said this with a wry smile on her face, and it took David a minute to recollect that he had been in an accident. "Oh my God! Did I hit anyone else?" he asked.

"From what I was told, you were pretty lucky and simply drove into the mountainside. There was a police car nearby and he radioed for an ambulance immediately. You've had an angioplasty, that's why your right wrist is sore and bruised. Your wife has been notified but I don't think she's come in yet. Now, relax. I need to check your IV and take another blood sample. Are you having any pain?"

Pain. It was nothing like the constricting, crushing agony he had experienced in the car but his chest ached as if he had done way too many bench-presses the previous day. *A heart attack! How could that be? Shit, I'm only forty-two. This can't be happening to me,* he thought.

"No, I don't really have any pain," he told Mary Ann. "But why would I have a heart attack? I've never had any health problems," he asked, incredulously.

"Dr. Schreiber is just making his rounds," she responded, "He is the cardiologist who opened up your plugged artery. He'll answer any questions you may have."

Markus Schreiber was a thirty-six-year-old cardiologist whose prematurely gray hair made him look ten years older than he was. A gold medalist in his medical class, he had become a red-hot resident in the cardiology program at the

University of British Columbia in Vancouver before accepting a fellowship in Interventional Cardiology at Harvard. He was now on staff at St. Luke's and also taught at the medical school. Schreiber was wearing a black long-sleeved tee shirt under his white lab coat. His casual appearance did not detract from his confident and professional manner.

"How are you feeling, David?" he asked matter-of-factly, glancing at a clipboard at the foot of the bed. "I'm Doctor Schreiber."

"I'm feeling okay, I guess, but I'm surprised to be here, doc. They say I've had a heart attack."

Dr. Schreiber flipped through David's chart. "Well, your heart was beating very irregularly to the extent that it was not pumping your blood properly any more. We checked your coronary arteries and found a blockage, which we were able to open up again for you. The procedure restored the blood flow to the damaged heart tissue. We'll still need to do an ultrasound of your heart and get you on a treadmill to see how your heart is functioning."

"But I'll be all right, won't I?" whispered David, He had never felt more vulnerable.

Schreiber hesitated. "Having one heart attack as you did more than quadruples your chance of having another one. We can reduce your risk by following current medication, diet, and exercise guidelines. You have already been started on a beta-blocker, which is a cardioprotective medication that lowers your blood pressure and heart rate. You will also be on a statin drug to lower cholesterol, along with an ACE inhibitor. These medications help to stabilize the plaque in your coronary arteries to reduce the risk of a subsequent heart attack. In addition, you are advised to take a low-dose aspirin every day for the rest of your life. For the next year after your angioplasty, you will also be taking an additional blood thinner to prevent clots from forming in your stent. We'll also get you to see a dietician and get you hooked up to our Cardiac Rehab program. You'll need to make some lifestyle changes, you know—quit smoking, get some exercise—that sort of thing. Although life expectancy following a single event is often diminished, it plummets dramatically after a subsequent episode," he stated frankly. "Our job is to prevent you from having another heart attack. Think of yourself as a twin-engine jet plane. You have just lost one engine and a little altitude, but you will still be able to fly. Lose another engine, my friend, and you'll be hooped."

David was proud of his near-photographic memory, but Schreiber's words had already faded. This was a frickin' nightmare. All he could think of was that he had been fine one minute, and the next a cardiac cripple, condemned to a life of being a prescription pill junkie and walking on a treadmill. "The follow-up can be done through your family doctor's office. We'll send him copies of the test results and the discharge summary," concluded the cardiologist.

David didn't have a family doctor. He had been in perfect health; the odd time he was feeling sick, he simply went to a local walk-in clinic.

"Thanks, doc," he mumbled, as Schreiber nodded and strode towards his next patient.

---

David spent three days in the ICU, and one by one his lines came out and he began to feel more human again. As he regained his strength he chatted with Mary Ann, who always seemed happy to pause for a moment in her work. She usually had an anecdote to share about her experiences as a nurse, and their brief conversations relieved the tedium of his hospital stay.

He was transferred to the step-down unit on the same floor as the ICU and remained connected to a telemetry unit, a machine that functions like a wireless ECG monitor. David had three room-mates, all of whom had cardiac problems. Although David was the youngest on the ward, he could see that this disease cut a swath across all walks of life.

Ken, a retired high school teacher who had emigrated from England, was sixty-eight years old and required a pacemaker because many years of high blood pressure and a heart attack had damaged the conducting system of his heart. Ken understood Dr. Schreiber's explanation of his condition, which he recounted to David. "Your electrical wires became frayed, and now the current does not flow through them properly, but we can fix that."

Chuck was a fifty-six-year-old firefighter recovering from bypass surgery after having suffered his second heart attack. David recalled Schreiber's stern warning that he needed to make significant changes in his life so that he would not become a "repeat offender."

Raj, a fifty-one-year-old, originally from Kenya, had been a security guard at the hospital for the last twelve years but was recently laid off when the health authority privatized many services as a cost-cutting measure. He had an enlarged heart and leaky valves, which had made his chest fill up with fluid. Dr. Schreiber had told him that heart valves are like doors, and if you slam one shut, it should close firmly against the door casing. The blood should not leak back through the valve but instead flow through the next valve to the appropriate chamber of the heart. Raj's valves, by contrast, had become like a saloon door, allowing the blood to flow in either direction.

David and his roommates, with little to do other than pass the time, found that they had much in common. They knew that they were the lucky ones, and that many people who have heart attacks do not make it to hospital. The four men shared their fears and plans for the future with each other and felt the closeness of brothers in arms, promising to stay in touch after they were discharged.

Schreiber was making his rounds. "Remember me, doc?" David greeted him. "I'm the jet plane that lost an engine."

"Of course, David. Your job now is to keep all your remaining cylinders firing. We'll do our part, and I hope you'll do yours. I discharged a gentleman yesterday who has now had his third heart attack and still refuses to give up alcohol and cigarettes. He's down to his last working cylinder and can't fly anymore, but I'm sure he'll still taxi over to the bar for refuelling," Schreiber said, milking his jet engine analogy for all it was worth.

The hospital dietician came by to visit. After overwhelming David with information on nutrition, she handed him some pamphlets to read on a healthy-heart diet. David stuffed them into the bedside drawer, recognizing that there was a wide gulf between the suggested guidelines and the restaurant meals he had with clients or the takeout food he ate at his apartment.

"Lunch time!" smiled the care aide as she delivered a tray to David's bedside. He removed the plastic lid from his plate revealing a white bun with a gray burger.

A long, limp slice of pickle garnished the top. There was a dollop of an amorphous orange substance along with something mushy and green that may have, at one time, been a vegetable. This was accompanied by a serving of orange juice in a translucent plastic container sealed with a foil lid, along with a cup of vanilla ice cream covered with a cardboard lid for dessert.

Unappealing as the food looked, David was hungry and in no mood to protest, "I'm back," he thought, as he dug into the burger.

---

David was a successful lawyer and proud that he had been made a partner at Kane Wallace & Sullivan in Vancouver. He had worked hard to get through law school, and had managed to get an articling position at the firm by volunteering to work in the office while he was a law student. It did not hurt that his father, a prominent judge, had put in a good word for him as well. David did not hide this fact. "You'd have to be an idiot not to leverage your connections," he'd admitted to his peers.

David was brighter than average and appeared to succeed through a combination of hard work, determination, and getting a few strings pulled at opportune times. This had been a good strategy for climbing the ladder at work, but he had to admit that the passive neglect of both his health and his marriage had taken their toll.

Jessica and the kids had been by earlier that day. Rebecca had made him a get-well card on the computer and Adam had given his father a copy of his latest soccer team trading card.

David had thought that he and Jessica were soul mates

when they had started dating in college. They had shared similar interests and had an overlapping circle of friends. With similar goals and desires, they had often known what the other was thinking. David had found that Jessica was easy to be with and rarely complained when he played hockey with the boys and then retreated to the bar afterwards. They had married after she had finished her degree in Education. She had taught full time until Rebecca was born. She had continued to teach half-time until two years later when Adam came along. At that point she devoted herself fully to her kids and household, as well as supporting David in his work. With David's long hours at the firm, especially while he was establishing himself, it seemed the ideal relationship. He was able to concentrate on work while Jessica managed everything else. Somewhere along the way, however, their relationship had become strained. David spent long days at the office, compounded by an increasing number of late night dinner meetings, leaving Jessica wondering why she had married a man she never saw. At one point she broke down and accused him of having an affair. David denied that allegation, but in retrospect he realized he had broken the PPF rule that Bishop Mahoney had taught them in marriage preparation class. The most important principle to follow in creating a long and happy marriage, he had said, is to "Put your Partner First." He argued that if all major decisions made in a marriage were seen through the lens of how it would affect the partner—and if those decisions honestly reflected the shared desire to put one's partner first—that the marriage would stand the test of time.

As he looked back on it, David realized that his relationship with Jessica had become more like "Every Man for

Himself"—each seeking to fulfill personal goals, objectives, and desires; the PPF motto had gone out the window. After all, when he worked hard all week, was it not more important that he go on a weekend hockey trip with his friends rather than accompany Jessica and the kids to her parents' home for a visit?

Their fights had become more frequent, followed by icy silences, until they had agreed that for the sake of the kids that they would spend some time apart and try to work things out.

Time apart meant a rented suite for David, but he wasn't sure when or how they were going to start working things out. He saw Rebecca and Adam on alternate weekends, and spent time driving them to soccer games and birthday parties, always feeling a little uncomfortable when he had to speak to the parents of their friends. He knew several other couples in the same situation, but it was certainly not what he had envisioned for himself when he was in law school, planning for his future.

In hindsight, he realized that he had been living the dream—a smart and pretty wife, two lovely children, an enviable job as partner of an important downtown firm, and a comfortable home complete with a tall cedar hedge and a golden retriever in a quiet residential neighbourhood. Without any apparent effort he had remained fit and healthy. How he yearned to go back to those halcyon days now.

In the hospital, Jessica had appeared concerned, and when he had reassured her that he would be fine she had looked suitably relieved. "When will you be able to go home?" she had asked.

"The cardiologist said tomorrow morning if my blood

pressure remains normal and if I pass my stress test and cardiac ultrasound. I think they want to kick me out because the hospital is chronically short of beds … just kidding … I really will be fine."

"I'm afraid I won't be able to drive you to your apartment tomorrow," said Jessica. "I have to work."

"Work? What do you mean?" He was slightly stunned by her announcement.

"I submitted my name for teacher-on-call, and I've accepted a job share position that opened up due to a maternity leave. Don't worry about the kids; it's only three days a week and Mom is eager to help out with their after school activities." Her parents did not live far from the family house, and relished the role of being active grandparents.

"Well … that's great, I guess," murmured David. "Congratulations."

There was an awkward pause, only broken when Rebecca and Adam announced that they were hungry and wanted something from the vending machine in the lobby. As usual, David nodded his agreement and Jessica shook her head disapprovingly. David reached for his wallet in the drawer beside his bed. It was just one of many small disagreements that had soured their relationship. He liked to buy the kids treats whenever he saw them, although Jessica had repeatedly accused him of poisoning them with junk food. This time Jessica's attitude irritated him even more than usual, and he insisted on giving the kids coins for the machine. As they left the hospital room, he felt an unexpected stab of self-pity, "Don't worry about me, I'll take a cab tomorrow," he whispered to Jessica's departing form.

# CHAPTER 2

*"We are what we repeatedly do.*
*Excellence, then, is not an act, but a habit."*

**Aristotle**
(384-322 BC) Greek Philosopher

David took a deep breath as he walked out of the hospital on a sunny morning. Looking towards the North Shore Mountains he realized, perhaps for the first time in his adult life, the meaning of the expression "glad to be alive." He knew that he had been given a reprieve and that he didn't intend to find himself in the ICU again anytime soon—or worse.

The cabbie stepped out of the car and opened the back door for David, who threw his bag on the back seat and climbed in after it. "Where can I take you, mate?" the cabbie asked him in a clipped British accent. David noticed that they were about the same age. His driver was of South Asian origin, with a slight, but athletic build. His pleasant smile and comfortable demeanour suggested to David that the man actually liked his job. David gave him the address of his Yaletown apartment and off they went.

As they crossed the Lions Gate Bridge, David peered at the sailboats on the sparkling water of Burrard Inlet, and the container ships making their way towards the Port of Vancouver. The majestic trees in Stanley Park stood tall, the popcorn and roasted nut vendors were out in full force on Beach Avenue, and all around people could be seen jogging, roller blading, or cycling along the Seawall.

At a stoplight, David noticed a small paperback book beside his bag on the back seat. Idly, David looked at the title: *12 Habits of Healthy People*. He thumbed through the book, which contained tips to improve health, along with some exercises and recipes. There was no indication who had written it, although the publisher was listed as the *Magna Vita Institute*.

"Is this your place, mate?" asked the driver as they pulled up to David's apartment. "Yes, thanks. Hey, I found this book on the seat. Do you know whom it belongs to?" inquired David as he got out his wallet.

"You're my first fare today. The book must have been left in the car yesterday," the driver said. As David handed him the book, a business card fell out. Listed on it was the name ***Sanjay Purewal, Magna Vita Institute***, along with a local phone number.

David said, "I don't mind phoning this guy and telling him he lost his book. Besides, it looks interesting, and it will give me something to read. The doctor doesn't want me to go back to work yet."

"All right, that's sorted then. Good luck," the driver replied, as he thanked David for his generous tip and waved good-bye.

.......................................................................

The apartment was a mess, but it was always a mess. David had been rushing to leave for Whistler, so had not put the dishes in the dishwasher, and had left clothes strewn around his bedroom. He threw his bag on his bed and opened the windows to let in some fresh air. The clean-up could wait; he felt tired and drained after his near-death experience. He was not in great shape to begin with, but now he was played out even after a minimal amount of exertion. He sat down on his sofa to flip through the booklet he had found.

*12 Habits of Healthy People* intrigued David. Was it some kind of weird coincidence, finding a book with a title like this one week after a heart attack? The introduction argued that if the reader wanted to have good health, and enjoy it in abundance, it was essential to develop these habits. It would be necessary to incorporate these behaviours into everyday life rather than making temporary changes. It would be challenging, but the rewards, promised the unknown author, would be true health, happiness, and harmony.

*Sounds like new-age mumbo jumbo*, thought David, but intuitively he felt that he needed to know this information, so he began reading.

*Health* implies far more than simply the "absence of disease or illness." Just as peace is more than the absence of war and conflict, joy is not just the absence of sorrow, and love is greater than the absence of hatred or indifference—so too is health more than the absence of disease. Good health may be hard to define, but we can easily recognize when it is absent.

Perhaps a negative definition can be useful as the Buddha simply defined Enlightenment as "the end of suffering." This does not spell out what enlightenment is or how it can be attained or set out a specific definition that may be too narrow or miss the mark; only that there will be an end of suffering on all levels. So too, health can be seen as "the end of illness"—in all its physical and psychological forms and dimensions.

*Health is a state of balance and harmony at all levels*—mental, physical, emotional, spiritual, social, and even financial. It is wholeness in its most profound sense; it exists when all the elements and forces making up an individual resonate in equilibrium. Recognize that health is a continuum, not an "all or none" phenomenon. Numerous factors may allow us to move from being a little healthy to enjoying more vigorous health. Good health, then, is a delicate homeostasis between factors that trigger illness and others that keep illness at bay. Fortunately, many of these factors are within our control! Choices we make, along with factors in our environment as well as our genetic predisposition, all influence our health. Psychosocial factors are also important in having good health. Strong connections to a spiritual reality as well as to family and community, along with meaningful work, all result in a high level of satisfaction that equates to better health outcomes.

When there is a departure from health, disease eventually occurs. To reduce our risk of disease it is prudent to make mindful choices in a proactive manner to optimize our health. As we are not able to alter several determinants of health, such as age and genetic background, we need to focus on lifestyle choices that we can control[1].

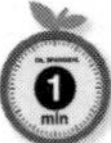

**One minute message**

The *majority* of premature deaths and age-related illnesses are preventable with *lifestyle modification* …

Most heart attacks, strokes, many cancers, obesity, diabetes, falls, fractures, infections, and many other illnesses can be *prevented* through proper diet, vigorous exercise, and other factors that are within our *control.*

---

[1] King, Dana, et al. 2007. Turning back the clock: Adopting a healthy lifestyle in middle age. *The American Journal of Medicine* 120: 598–603. Adopting a healthy lifestyle (diet, exercise, non-smoking) in middle aged subjects (45-64 yrs) resulted in a prompt reduction in cardiovascular disease and mortality.

“It is critical to integrate these changes into our lives rather than thinking of them as temporary measures adopted to achieve only one specific goal such as weight reduction. Consequently, these patterns of behaviour must become habits. The word “habit” comes from the Latin “habitus,” signifying the indwelling presence and operation of these behaviours that reflect one's condition or character. In English, the word “habitus” refers to one's body build and constitution, especially as it relates to predisposition to disease.

The stages involved in learning new skills follow a predictable sequence. Initially, one does not have any idea what skills need to be mastered. This stage is called *unconsciously incompetent.* This may apply to serving a ball in tennis, making a chip shot in golf, a turn-around jump shot in basketball, getting through a slalom course on a water ski, or making lifestyle choices that can improve health and vitality.

Once we are aware of what we want to do, we realize that we do not understand the fundamentals of how to do it. In this stage we are *consciously incompetent.* From here, learning can occur. If courses are taken and instruction is given, *explicit (conscious) learning* happens. Alternately, if someone practises and gets better without being aware of exactly what they are doing, *implicit (unconscious) learning* has occurred. In either case, through practice, repetition, and feedback one now becomes *consciously competent.* When learning new skills, one needs to mechanically go through the motions, slowly and deliberately, step by step, thinking about what it is that we want to do. When a skill or behaviour is so ingrained that it occurs automatically, after thousands of backhand shots, for example, so that we are able to perform the desired task instinctively, no longer thinking about ourselves or what we need to do—we are *unconsciously competent.* At this point the dancer becomes the dance. We are fully engaged, with no fear of failure; enjoying peak performance by living in the moment. For athletes this is sometimes called being in the "zone." We can also state that at this point, the behaviour has become a *habit.*

---

This was making sense to David. He realized that some of his habits were destructive and had led to his premature admission to a coronary care unit. Maybe this was his opportunity to develop some more positive habits. He certainly was not in the mood to clean up his apartment, so he decided to read on.

*Let food be your medicine;*
*and medicine be your food.*

**Hippocrates**
(460-377 BC) Greek Physician

---

## HABIT ONE: DIET

The first and most fundamental step to a healthy life is to maintain a healthy diet. The statement "you are what you eat" is, in fact, a truism. Just as the construction of a quality home requires superior building products and skilled workers, so too is the body's health and vitality dependent on the foods that supply it with the required building blocks.

It is critical, therefore, to be selective in the food choices we make, as these provide the raw materials that become incorporated into our bodies. Unlike quality homes, however, our bodies are alive, so our cells—the timbers and bricks we are made of—are constantly being replaced and exchanged. We consume nutrients for the manufacture, replacement, and maintenance of living cells that form the structural elements of our bodies: skin, muscles, connective tissue, bones, and organs, as well as functional elements such as hormones, digestive enzymes, neurotransmitters, and antibodies.

Building blocks can be divided into *macronutrients* and *micronutrients*. Macronutrients are foods from which we derive calories (energy) and include protein, carbohydrates, and fats. Micronutrients do not provide the body with energy but with factors necessary for proper cellular and organ functions. These include vitamins and minerals such as iron, calcium, magnesium, zinc, and copper. There are also minerals required in such miniscule amounts that they are often referred to *as trace elements*. Although tiny in quantity they are vitally important as they enable the body to produce enzymes, hormones, and other substances essential for proper growth and development. Furthermore, there are thousands of phytochemicals or plant-derived substances (in supplement form they are often called neutraceuticals indicating that they are naturally occurring substances that produce a physiological effect), which function as antioxidants or chemicals that inhibit the growth of micro-tumours, which are constantly forming in our bodies. The full role of these micronutrients and the amounts required is not precisely known. It is prudent to take in a large variety of fresh whole foods to increase the likelihood of absorbing these micronutrients in sufficient quantities. Try to buy foods that are in season and be adventuresome in seeking out different foods. In addition to these nutrients, fibre is another important component of a healthy diet. Fibre is either soluble (turns to gel when water is added) or insoluble. Both types are indigestible and provide no nutritional value to the diet, but are essential in adding bulk and moisture to the stool to assist evacuation.

When living cells are no longer able to function, they die and need to be removed and replaced. This is a process known as *necrosis* and is mostly seen when tissue is injured or infected. But cells also undergo a process of programmed cell death called *apoptosis*. In this case, the cell dies cleanly and the components are broken down and reused without "rotting" as is the case with necrosis. Through this process, tissues remain vital and functioning optimally. In this way, there is a continuous renewal happening in our bodies; cells are broken down and new cells are generated. Think of hedges being pruned in the spring to make them more vigorous and allow new growth to occur.

Interestingly, cancer cells seem to have lost this property of apoptosis, returning to their ancestral "every man for himself" philosophy and proliferating their own cell line to the detriment of the organism as a whole[2].

Normally apoptosis occurs in approximately one hundred billion cells per day. This is the equivalent of the entire body replacing itself every eighteen to twenty-four months. Many tissues replace themselves at a slower rate, but some, like the lining of the intestines and the skin, do so much more quickly[3].

The raw materials that the body needs are termed *essential nutrients. The body requires them but cannot make them. Therefore, they need to be obtained from the diet.* These include: essential amino acids, the building blocks of proteins; essential fatty acids, carbohydrates, vitamins and minerals.

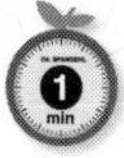

**One minute message**

Wholesome foods are the cornerstone to good health.

Eat from the *rainbow*. Enjoy intensely coloured, unprocessed foods—as our grandparents used to eat—with little added and little taken away.

The key to good nutrition is getting enough beneficial food into your body, and reducing the amount of harmful food. The framework is a simple one.

---

[2] These characteristics of cancer cell growth are discussed in more detail in "Foods that Fight Cancer," Chapter 2: "What is Cancer?" (see Reference section).

[3] Israels, 1999. Apoptosis. *Stem Cell*: 17(5) 306–3 as quoted by Dr. Aileen Burford-Mason in a workshop entitled "Wellness from within: Nutrition and the mind-body connection" presented at the conference "When the Body Forgets to Heal" May 27–29, 2005 Victoria, BC, Canada.

**Eat more:**

1. Unprocessed, unrefined, whole, and raw foods, including fruits and vegetables with intense colours.
2. Healthy fats: Omega-3 fatty acid sources (oily fish—such as salmon and sardines, and oily nuts and seeds—such as flax, hemp, chia, and walnuts).
3. Probiotics; helpful bacteria in cultured foods: yogurt, kefir, sauerkraut, etcetera.

**Eat less:**

1. Processed foods high in sugar, salt, and fat. Reduce processed carbohydrates (high glycemic index foods and "white foods").
2. Hydrogenated oils (trans fatty acids), found in prepared and fried foods.
3. Animal foods, high in protein and saturated fats (meats and dairy).

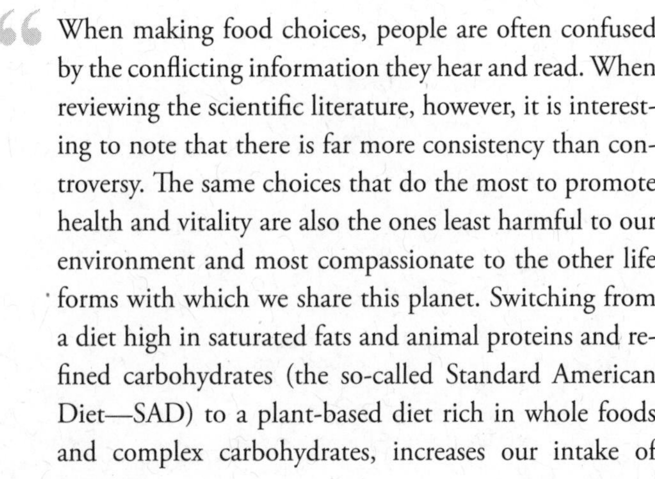

" When making food choices, people are often confused by the conflicting information they hear and read. When reviewing the scientific literature, however, it is interesting to note that there is far more consistency than controversy. The same choices that do the most to promote health and vitality are also the ones least harmful to our environment and most compassionate to the other life forms with which we share this planet. Switching from a diet high in saturated fats and animal proteins and refined carbohydrates (the so-called Standard American Diet—SAD) to a plant-based diet rich in whole foods and complex carbohydrates, increases our intake of protective food substances and reduces our intake of disease promoting substances.[4] This same diet reduces the incidence of obesity, Type 2 diabetes, heart disease, stroke, sexual dysfunction, cancer, arthritis, osteoporosis, Alzheimer's disease, and depression.[5] Similarly, it promotes optimal health, vitality at every level, happiness, global nutrition and sustainability, and so perhaps even world peace!

It is unfortunate that modern society focuses mainly on food for enjoyment and fuel—only a necessary replenishment of energy delivered fast and cheap, without concern for its impact on nourishing our organ systems. This disconnect between what we eat and what is healthy to eat is largely responsible for the sharp increase in the occurrence of diseases such as diabetes, heart disease, and cancer, which only a century ago were relatively rare. The fact that this marked increase in these diseases (cancer in particular) comes at a time when medical science has never been more robust is alarming indeed[6].

---

[4] Robbins, John, 2001, *The Food Revolution, How Your Diet can Help Save Your Life and the World.* Foreword by Dean Ornish, MD, Conari Press, Berkeley, California. This thoughtful and well researched book outlines the perils of many of today's foods and gives compelling evidence for healthier alternatives.

[5] Lie, Désirée, October 12, 2009, Mediterranean Diet May Cut Depression Risk, *Medscape Education Clinical Briefs*. Following a diet high in vegetables, nuts, olive oils and unprocessed grains was found to lower the risk of depression by 30 percent.

[6] Béliveau, Richard; Gingras, Denis, 2007, *Cooking with Foods that Fight Cancer*, McClelland and Stewart, Toronto, page 99.

He was startled by his ringing telephone. David's mother, not surprisingly, wanted to know how he was feeling and told him she had spoken to her family physician about seeing David as a patient. As it turned out, a new doctor was joining the group and taking some new patients. She had set up an appointment for him the day after tomorrow. He would be seeing Dr. Osler at 3:45 PM. *Well, that was Step One*, thought David as he hung up. Dr. Schreiber had advised him to follow-up with his family doctor, and now it looked as if he might have one.

David was too tired to read further, but the book's premise that he could influence his health by simple choices had made an impact on him. It might explain, too, why he had suffered his heart attack in the first place—and why society in general is so vulnerable to preventable diseases.

He decided to forego the greasy fast food to which he had become accustomed since he had moved out of the family home, and instead called up an associate from his firm to suggest they meet for dinner at a local restaurant.

Joanna Lee had studied law at Osgoode Hall in Toronto but had moved back to Vancouver three years ago. Like David, she had managed to get an articling position at Kane Wallace & Sullivan. Unlike David, her father was not a judge, and her success was based on sheer hard work and determination. Joanna had recently been working on several of the same files as David.

At the Bistro Aubergine, David, mindful of what he had just been reading, ordered poached spring salmon with wild mushroom risotto and Caesar salad. Joanna had the roasted butternut squash soup and arugula salad with fresh figs, goat cheese, and a port wine reduction. They sipped a glass of red wine as David told her about his heart attack and that he would not be in the office for at least the next few weeks. He was amazed at the freshness and tastiness of the food, especially after the blandness of his recent hospital fare, and wondered whether he would even have noticed before his heart attack.

Geoff Sullivan, a founding partner of the firm had visited David in hospital and told him to take all the time he needed. They had managed to postpone one of his cases that was going to trial, and there were enough lawyers in the firm that they could cover him while he was away. Joanna was prepared to work on his files and phone or e-mail David for his input as needed.

Although he felt capable of driving, David's car had been badly damaged in the accident, and the insurance company had yet to decide whether it was worth repairing or whether they would write it off. Besides, Dr. Schreiber had told him no driving or sex for at least two weeks, until he was reassessed by his family doctor. He had almost chuckled out loud when he had been told this, as he knew he would be able to adhere to the second recommendation all too easily. He also felt that while he was recuperating he could certainly manage without a car. He accepted Joanna's offer to drive him home from the restaurant. It was a wonderful feeling to lie in his own bed after being in hospital, and as he went to sleep he felt like an incredibly fortunate man.

David slept a lot longer than the nurses would have let him. The hospital had supplied him with his medications for the first two days, but now he needed to get his prescriptions filled.

After his shower, he thought about making some bacon and eggs, but then he remembered the book's recommendation to avoid saturated fats. He opted for a bowl of oatmeal instead, adding raisins, brown sugar, and cinnamon for good measure.

After breakfast, he sat down with a cup of tea and reread the list of three things to eat more of and three things to eat less of. It sounded simple enough, but he didn't like the thought of giving up meat. Did the author mean he would have to become vegetarian? And what was a glycemic index? Or hydrogenated vegetable oil? That was a plant oil, so it should be good, right? And more importantly, was this kind of diet going to help him to shed the twenty pounds he needed to lose? Or reduce his risk of having another heart attack?

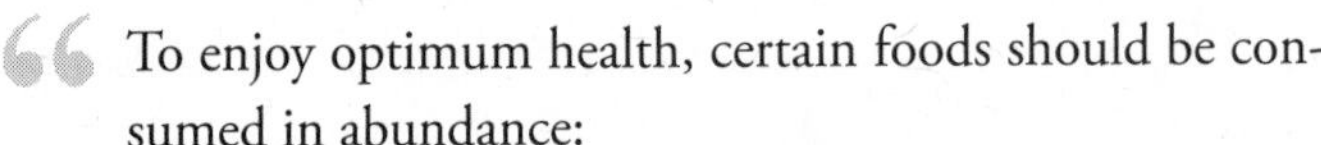

To enjoy optimum health, certain foods should be consumed in abundance:

**1. Eat more unprocessed, unrefined, whole, and raw foods.** In particular, choose whole grains, which provide various vitamins, minerals, phytochemicals, and other bioactive components that work together synergistically to confer health benefits. There is evidence that regular consumption of whole grain products (such as wheat, barley, oats, buckwheat, quinoa, kamut, spelt, and rye) can lower the risk of cardiovascular disease, diabetes, and cancer, and can help maintain a healthy weight. When possible, choose organically-grown foods. There is growing evidence that organically grown foods contain more nutrients, in particular micronutrients, such as minerals and bioflavonoids. These bioflavonoids are found in brightly coloured foods and may also reduce the risk of cardiovascular disease as well as cancer and other diseases.

For example, *lycopene* from tomatoes is associated with a lower risk of prostate cancer. Lycopene is more concentrated in tomato paste and sauces compared to fresh tomatoes. *Lutein*, also from red and orange coloured fruits and vegetables, can protect against macular degeneration (a form of eye disease that can lead to blindness). *Anthocyanidins* from blueberries are antioxidants that may also reduce macular degeneration. *Sulphoraphanes* from broccoli inhibit a bacterium associated with ulcers and stomach cancer. And *resveratrol*, from red wine, grapes, and other pigmented fruits is helpful in the treatment of coronary artery disease, because it acts as an antioxidant, is anti-inflammatory, inhibits platelet aggregation, and causes blood-vessel dilatation. It also appears to inhibit the formation of cancerous cells. Therefore, eating a plate full of richly coloured foods; dark green, red, orange, and blue, ensures that the diet will contain these beneficial substances. Taking several foods in combination results in a synergistic increase in the absorption of antioxidants and other nutrients compared to taking the foods individually.

Early results show that combining foods can offer even greater cancer prevention and overall healthier combinations of nutrients than any one food can offer individually. Salmon, watercress, broccoli florets, and walnuts combine numerous cancer fighting ingredients, in particular, sulphoraphane and selenium. The combination of these two nutrients is 13 times more effective than either one alone. The *sulphoraphane* found in broccoli also has a synergistic relationship with lycopene (tomatoes) and with another *flavonoid*, apigenin, found in apples, beans, cherries, leeks, onions, barley. Eating meals that combine foods of different colors may also impart improved health benefits over eating any one colour of food alone.[7]

Berries, in particular, seem to be precious little gems. Cranberries, blueberries, blackberries, black currants, bilberries, and the Brazilian *açai* berry contain different combinations of health benefits, but generally they are rich in vitamins (particularly C), *flavonoids* such as quercetin and anthocyanin, fibre, and folic acid. They also appear to have some of the highest antioxidant levels of any foods.

In a study of Finnish men, those who ate 100 grams of frozen berries daily had 32–51 percent higher blood levels of quercetin—widely regarded as a cancer-preventing flavonoid as well as a substance shown to reduce symptoms of hay fever.[8]

Bioflavonoids are part of a large group of micronutrients known as anti-oxidants. Antioxidants are like rust inhibitors in the body. Apples that have been cut open turn brown when exposed to air due to oxidation. If apple slices are dipped in lemon juice (rich in an *antioxidant* called ascorbic acid or Vitamin C) they do not brown as quickly. In the body, antioxidants neutralize the harmful

---

[7] Heber, D. 2004. Vegetables, fruits and phytoestrogens in the prevention of diseases. *Journal of Postgraduate Medicine* 50(2): 145–149.

[8] Erlund, I., et al. 2003. Consumption of black currants, lingonberries and bilberries increases serum quercetin concentrations. *European Journal of Clinical Nutrition*, 57(1): 37–42.

"oxidative" effects of free radicals.

Biochemically, *free radicals* are any atoms or molecules that have a single unpaired electron in an outer shell. They can be formed when oxygen interacts with certain molecules. These highly unstable substances can be formed by the immune system to defend against viruses and bacteria. Tissue damage from the ingestion of toxins and exposure to radiation, including ultraviolet radiation is largely responsible for their formation. Cigarette smoke and other forms of air pollution result in free radical production that damages the lungs and leads to asthma, emphysema, and lung cancer.

Once formed these highly reactive radicals can start a chain reaction, like dominoes, leaving cellular destruction in their wake. The chief danger comes from the damage they can do when they react with important cellular components such as DNA, or the cell membrane. Cells may function poorly or die when this occurs. If not neutralized, this damage contributes to neurodegenerative conditions such as Parkinson's disease and Alzheimer's dementia as well as cancers, heart disease, and strokes. Even aging itself is possibly due to free radical damage. To reduce free radical damage the body has developed an elaborate defense system that is bolstered by antioxidants.

Antioxidants are molecules that can safely interact with free radicals and terminate the chain reaction before vital molecules are damaged. Although there are several enzyme systems within the body that scavenge free radicals, the principal micronutrient (vitamin) antioxidants are vitamin E, beta-carotene, and vitamin C. Additionally, selenium, a trace metal that is required for proper function of one of the body's antioxidant enzyme systems, is sometimes included in this category. The body cannot manufacture any of these micronutrients so they must be supplied in the diet.

While there is good evidence for the antioxidant effect of certain nutrients, some studies on the use of antioxidants have been disappointing and others have been inconclusive. For example, several early studies demonstrated that people who had high blood levels of beta carotene had a lower risk of heart disease and cancer. This fuelled the supplement market and soon beta carotene pills were being gobbled up by health-conscious consumers worldwide. Further studies demonstrated that the use of beta carotene supplements in isolation was not helpful and possibly even harmful to smokers, who are obviously at higher risk of poor health outcomes already. As it turns out, those people who had higher blood levels of beta carotene were more health conscious to begin with; they ate a diet rich in fruits and vegetables and were more likely to also be following a healthy lifestyle in terms of exercising and abstaining from smoking. So it was not surprising that they would enjoy better health outcomes. The beta carotene levels were simply a marker of this lifestyle. To believe that all these benefits could be obtained by taking a pill was an example of reductionist thinking—looking for short cuts and easy solutions.

Therefore, from a public health perspective, it is premature to make recommendations regarding antioxidant supplements and disease prevention. Perhaps the best advice, which comes from several authorities in cancer prevention, is to eat at least "five servings of fresh fruits or vegetables per day.

By consuming whole foods we can be certain that we are getting a combination of potent anti-oxidants into our bodies. In addition, combinations of anti-oxidants are synergistic. That means that eating several brightly-coloured fruits and vegetables together is better than eating just one. Washing such a meal down with flavonoid-rich green tea and finishing the meal with dark chocolate enhances the antioxidant effect even further. Good sources of these disease fighting micronutrients can be found in many richly coloured fruits, especially berries, beans, vegetables, whole grains, and spices.[9]

Besides selecting foods carefully, it is also important to find out where your food comes from. Locally grown foods are typically lower in preservatives as they do not need to travel great distances. They also require less storage and transportation costs and thus have a lighter environmental impact. Organic farming, in particular, is gentle and sustainable on the land and maintains intact ecosystems. Paradoxically, farms that use the highest levels of toxic pesticides do not have the least amount of pests on their crops. Much like overuse of antibiotics selects for resistant strains of bacteria, so too does the heavy use of pesticides lead to resistance in the very insects that the farmers are hoping to control. Poisoned insects poison birds and so

---

[9] Wu, X., et.al., 2004. Lipophilic and hydrophilic antioxidant capacities of common foods in the United States. *Journal of Agricultural and Food Chemistry* Jun 16, 52(12): 4026–4037. In this study the antioxidant content of more than 100 different foods was analyzed. Cranberries, blueberries, and blackberries were found to be the highest fruit sources; beans (red, kidney, pinto, and black varieties), artichokes, and russet potatoes the best vegetable sources; and pecans, walnuts, and hazelnuts the best nut sources. Although they are usually consumed in small amounts, ground cloves, ground cinnamon, and oregano were the spices found to be highest in antioxidants.

on up the food chain. Organically produced foods are increasingly available and will be produced more economically as consumer demand increases. Make an effort to support organic farms and local farmers' markets whenever possible.

It is also important to consume an abundance of *raw fruits and vegetables*, as several nutrients, in particular, *enzymes*, are destroyed by cooking. Enzymes are required for the optimal digestion and absorption of foods as well as for numerous cellular functions. Their exclusion can result in multiple adverse health consequences. Juicing is an efficient way of extracting nutrients from raw foods such as greens by reducing most of the indigestible cellulose.

**2. Eat more foods containing essential fatty acids**. When considering dietary fats, do not think high fat vs. low fat foods, but rather bad fats vs. good fats. Fats contain more calories, that is, yield more energy per gram than carbohydrates and proteins. This is neither good nor bad, but should be accounted for when determining serving size. Fats that are required by the body but not manufactured in the body are called *essential fatty acids*. These are required for the synthesis of cell walls and as building blocks for many of the body's hormones and neurotransmitters. Fat is required for proper development and function of the brain and eyes just as protein is required for muscles, carbohydrates for fuel and calcium for bones.

Fat molecules can be classified by how many carbon atoms they contain and by how many hydrogen ions are bound to them. When hydrogen is bound to every available carbon atom this is called a *saturated fat* and these are harder fats mostly of animal origin (like butter and lard). When one carbon site is not bound with a hydrogen atom, this is called a *monounsaturated fat* (avocados and olive oil are rich in these) or *polyunsaturated fatty acids* (PUFA) when multiple carbon sites are unbound. Unsaturated fats can be further classified by how the hydrogen ions bind to the carbon atom. If they are bound on the same side of the carbon chain, this is called a cis-isomer and when bound on opposite sides it is a trans-isomer. So *trans fats* are unsaturated fatty acids (monounsaturated or PUFA) in the trans-isomer form that may be naturally occurring, but are mostly synthetically formed. It turns out that these are very unhealthy fats and need to be avoided. (Trans fats will be discussed in more detail shortly.) Depending on the chemical structure of PUFAs they are classified as omega-3, omega-6, and omega-9. Omega-9 fatty acids (FA) are synthesized from other fatty acids and are therefore not absolutely required in the diet. Both omega-3 and omega-6 FA are essential for good health and need to be supplied in the diet.

Omega-6 fatty acids are necessary for normal growth and development of cell membranes, especially for skin, hair, and bones as well as brain function. Omega-6 FAs are precursors for prostaglandins and other biologically active molecules which help maintain the reproductive system. Sources of omega-6 FAs include poultry, eggs, nuts, most vegetable oils and oil seeds such as canola, sunflower, soybean, and cottonseed oils. An important omega-6 FA helpful for eczema and other skin conditions is gamma linolenic acid (GLA), found in evening primrose oil, borage oil, and black currant oil.

Whereas omega-3 FAs reduce inflammation, excess omega-6 FAs promote inflammation and contribute to arthritis, asthma, atherosclerosis, blood clotting, tumour growth, and depression. Both omega-3 and omega-6 fatty acids were similarly abundant in the diet several generations ago. However, farming practices and processing of foods have resulted in a relative deficiency of omega-3 FAs to the extent that most diets now contain ten to twenty times more omega-6 content than omega-3. This is why it is so important to make the effort to get enough omega-3s in the diet and through supplements. A diet rich in omega-3 fatty acids can be part of an *"anti-inflammatory diet."* Avoidance of refined carbohydrates and an abundance of whole grains and omega-3-fatty-acid rich foods have been shown to reduce inflammation in joints and blood vessels. In addition, turmeric, ginger, garlic, kelp, shiitake mushrooms, blueberries, broccoli, green tea, papayas, and other richly pigmented fruits and vegetables all have an anti-inflammatory effect.

Sources of omega-3 fatty acids include whole grains, especially flax, chia, and hemp, nuts—particularly walnuts—and soy beans, along with wild oily fish such as salmon, sardines, herring, mackerel, and anchovies. The omega-3 FAs that the human body requires are long carbon-chain omega-3s called EPA and DHA (eicosapentaenoic acid and docosahexaenoic acid). These are found in fish but can also be synthesized from the shorter omega-3 FA, alpha-linolenic acid (ALA) which is found in nuts and seeds. The problem is that the conversion to the necessary long-chain FAs may be as low as 5 percent and is reduced by many factors, including the presence of sugar, alcohol, trans fats, and also viral illnesses[10]. Therefore, ideally, direct sources of DHA should be part of a healthy diet.

Higher levels of omega-3 FAs, DHA in particular, have been found helpful for multiple conditions and are one of the most evidence-based supplements for all age groups. DHA supplements have now been added to prenatal vitamins and infant formulas, as they promote better development of the brain and eyes and may keep infants happier and more content. Interestingly, the same omega-3 supplements that benefit newborns may reduce post-partum depression in mothers, and depressive disorders in general. In addition, essential fatty acids may help improve concentration and have been used to treat attention deficit disorder.

Fish oil supplements are also helpful to reduce inflammation and are often recommended for swollen and painful joints whether from sports or arthritis.

The oils are widely used to improve cholesterol levels in patients with a history or risk factors for heart disease. Because of their multiple benefits, they may be more helpful to improve overall health and have less adverse effects than many prescription medications used to treat heart disease. Depending on risk factors and lipid levels, however, prescription medications are obviously still

[10] Michael-Titus, Adina T. 2009. Omega-3 fatty acids: Their neuroprotective and regenerative potential in traumatic neurological injury. Clinical Lipidology 4(3):343--353.

required for many people.

Because the composition of the brain is approximately 60 percent fats (largely DHA and EPA) fish consumption and fish oil supplements are also used in the elderly to reduce cognitive decline. By extension, they may be useful brain food for people of all ages.

There is little that can be done after a traumatic brain injury other than wait and hope for improvement. In fact, even one significant traumatic brain injury (concussion) resulting in a loss of consciousness with amnesia—commonly seen in sports injuries or car accidents—may increase the risk of neurodegenerative conditions (memory loss, Parkinson's disease, and Alzheimer's dementia) twenty or more years later. However, essential fatty acids, DHA in particular, have been found to aid in recovery and improve outcomes.

In addition to saving brain cells, the DHA fatty acids have been shown to reduce the risk of a leading cause of blindness. Age-related macular degeneration (AMD) is an incurable degenerative disease of the eyes; specifically the part of the retina in which the visual cells are most concentrated (the "macula") and which is therefore the most important for vision. The only effective treatment is prevention: wearing sunglasses that block UV light, avoiding smoking, maintaining a normal blood pressure and lean body weight, and eating a diet rich in antioxidant foods as well as the omega-3 fatty acids EPA and DHA. The antioxidant vitamins C and E, the pro-vitamin A; beta-carotene, zinc, and the plant derived bioflavonoids lutein and zeaxanthin are all protective. Omega-3 fatty acids defend against AMD by inhibiting inflammation, repairing oxidative damage, and suppressing the formation of abnormal blood vessels in the retina.[11]

While many health-conscious consumers avoid seafood products because of high mercury levels in some fish, it should be noted that fish oil capsules are distilled and therefore free of heavy metal contamination. In addition, small fish from cold waters such as sardines and salmon are generally low in mercury compared to larger tropical game fish.

Specific plant oils have recently been approved by Health Canada to be labelled as helpful in lowering cholesterol levels. Plant sterols (or stanols—and β-sitosterol in particular) are found in vegetable oils such as corn oil, wheat germ, canola oil, olive oil, as well as numerous grains, fruits, and vegetables. They have a similar biochemical structure to cholesterol (only found in animals) and are required for cell wall permeability and several biological functions. It has been shown that adding these plant oils to the diet can lower the harmful LDL cholesterol.[12]

**3. Eat more healthy bacteria.** Bacteria are single-celled organisms that inhabit our bodies by the billions. Harmful bacteria are certainly a cause of infection and illness,

---

[11] SanGiovanni, J.P., Chew E.Y., 2005. The role of omega-3 long-chain polyunsaturated fatty acids in health and disease of the retina. *Progress in Retina and Eye Research*, Jan; 24(1): 87-138. (Quoted by Dr. Kevin Parkinson, ophthalmologist, at the Coast Mountain Summit—Family Medicine Update, April 10, 2010, Whistler, BC, Canada). Omega-3 fatty acids found in fatty fish such as sardines and salmon may protect against progression of age-related macular degeneration (AMD), but the benefits appear to depend on the stage of the disease and whether certain supplements are taken, report researchers at Tufts University.

[12] Health Canada, 2010. Taking in 2g/day of plant sterols lowered LDL cholesterol by 8.8 percent based on 84 randomized controlled trials reviewed by Health Canada. "Plant Sterols and Cholesterol Lowering" *Bureau of Nutritional Sciences, Food Directorate, Health Canada*, May 2010.

and there is evidence that bacterial infection may have a causative role in many chronic conditions such as asthma, rheumatoid arthritis, and coronary artery disease. However, most of the bacteria in our bodies aid in the digestion of foods and assimilation of nutrients. Abundant amounts of healthy bacteria may also inhibit the harmful bacteria and therefore reduce risk of illness. Societies consuming a significant amount of cultured foods seem to enjoy greater health and longevity. The healthy bacteria are called *probiotics* and are found in cultured dairy products such as yogurt, kefir, buttermilk, and sour cream, as well as sauerkraut. These fermented foods increase seratonin and dopamine levels in the brain boosting alertness and making inclusion of these items a good choice for breakfast.

While "probiotics" are readily available in tablet form, these products may not contain the quality or quantity of helpful bacteria that they claim. This is another example of where it may be preferable to obtain the sought after nutrients in their whole food form, rather than in a supplement.[13] Healthy bacteria are also found on the skins of fruits and vegetables. This is a good reason to consume the peels of apples, pears, peaches, potatoes, carrots, and other produce. Foods that have not been sprayed with pesticides will naturally have a greater number of probiotics available. In addition to improving intestinal flora and digestion, probiotics can reduce bladder infections, and cholesterol levels, as well as boost

[13] Huff, Brenda, 2004, Caveat emptor, "Probiotic" may not be what they seem, *Canadian Family Physician* 50: 583–587.

immune function and reduce the risk of colon cancer.[14] Beneficial bacteria as well as enzymes are lost by cooking and processing. This is why it is vital to include plenty of fresh (raw) fruits and veggies in your daily diet.

In addition to killing the targeted harmful bacteria, antibiotics destroy billions of friendly bacteria leading to indigestion, diarrhea, and yeast infections. A particularly dangerous infection often seen in hospitals is due to a bug called Clostridium difficile. This bacterium—virtually only seen after the use of broad spectrum antibiotics—can cause severe colitis that may prove fatal. By ensuring a steady intake of probiotics (especially when antibiotics have been prescribed) some of the unwanted and potentially devastating effects of antibiotics may be mitigated. Interestingly, better attendance in the workplace has been correlated in one study to workers consuming probiotics in yogurt regularly.[15]

**One minute message**

There are *good fats* and *bad fats.*

Harmful fats promote obesity, diabetes, heart disease, dementia, and cancer. Healthy fats play an anti-inflammatory role and are protective.

Eat more fish as well as oily nuts and seeds and grains, such as flax, hemp, walnuts, almonds, chia seeds, and olive oil.

---

[14] Béliveau, Richard, 2005, *Foods That Fight Cancer*, McClelland and Stewart, Toronto, Canada

[15] Tubelius, P., et.al., 2005, Increasing work-place healthiness with the probiotic Lactobacillus reuteri: A randomised, double-blind placebo-controlled study. *Environmental Health* Nov 7, 4(1): 25.

“When consuming more of the foods that are beneficial to our health, we will automatically eat less food of lower quality that may be harmful. Specifically, there are foods one must avoid or minimize.

**1. Eat fewer processed foods in general and refined carbohydrates in particular**. Commercially prepared foods are intended to be appealing to a majority of consumers. They typically have a soft mouth feel because they are easy to chew and high in fat, and are often high in sugar and salt. A small amount of salt is essential for most animals including humans. Hence, terms like “she is the salt of the earth” emerged centuries ago. And ranchers still put salt blocks out for their cattle. Because salt used to be in short supply, our bodies became very efficient in reusing dietary salt. However, now our food is so heavily salted that the high sodium content increases the risk of high blood pressure leading to strokes, heart disease, kidney failure, and dementia. A vast majority of adults exceed upper daily limits for sodium, and even small children are getting too much, with one-to-eight-year-olds consuming more than twice the recommended adequate daily intake of 1,000 to 1,200 mg. of sodium per day.

New research shows sodium causes high blood pressure and damage to blood vessels in children, setting them up for an increased risk of stroke and heart disease later in life. Few people realize how much salt is added to grocery items by the food industry. About 80 percent of the salt in our diets is hidden; it comes from the processing of foods so consumers are less aware that it's there.

Grains are seeds that are very nutrient-dense as they are

intended to reproduce an entire plant. Whole grains contain the bran, germ, and endosperm, all of which contain specific nutrients. White flour is produced by removing the bran and the germ and milling the endosperm. The resulting powder is devoid of fibre and many of the nutrients found in whole grain. Several vitamins are then added back, creating a product that is then called "enriched" white flour. (This is like being robbed at gunpoint and told to hand over all of your money as well as your clothes; then the assailant returns your socks and underwear as well as bus fare, leaving you "enriched"!) "Whole wheat" flour is not much better; flour is flour and has a high *glycemic index* (see below). If you have inherited the genetic predisposition to easily turn food into fat, and if you do not burn all of the calories that you consume, be very prudent in the consumption of any baked goods where flour of any kind is the main ingredient.

*Fibre* is another important nutrient, although it does not provide the body with energy or enzymes needed for cellular function. Soluble fibres are those that become gelatinous when water is added. Insoluble fibres do not. Both are important to add bulk to stool and are essential to maintain a healthy colon. Gelatinous foods, such as chia seeds, high in soluble fibres, help to absorb toxins and bile acids and excrete them from the body. Fibre also helps to slow the absorption of carbohydrates resulting in a smoother delivery of energy to the body. Aim for 30–50 grams of fibre a day. This can be easily achieved by eating an abundance of fresh fruits and vegetables (particularly legumes) as well as nuts and whole grains. At the same time, avoid foods devoid of fibre such as starchy or "white" foods, including white flour, white rice, sugar, soft pasta, mashed potatoes, and "puffed" grain products made of refined wheat, rice, or corn.

The amount that carbohydrates have been processed is expressed on a scale called the glycemic index. The *glycemic index* (GI) refers to how quickly a food is converted into *glycogen* which is the form of sugar that is used as fuel by the body. The higher the GI the more rapidly the food can be absorbed and utilized. Furthermore, the higher the GI, the greater its effect on insulin secretion. This is why refined foods increase the risk of developing diabetes.[16] Processed foods generally have a higher GI than unprocessed foods. For example, fruit juices are higher than whole fruit, and flour is higher than whole grains. Check online for tables listing the GI of various foods. Examples are provided of high GI foods that need to be reduced and low GI foods that can be consumed in greater quantities without raising blood sugar levels.

A broader way of looking at blood sugars and diabetic risk is to consider the *glycemic load* (GL). This is akin to looking at the glycemic index of your whole dinner rather than just one item. The GL measures the total glycemic response from the type and amount of food consumed. It takes into account that eating high fibre fruits and vegetables along with proteins and fats lowers the absorption of high GI foods and therefore slows the entry of carbohydrates into the blood stream. Foods that keep the GL of a meal low result in a slower rate of

[16] Hodge, A. M., et.al., 2004 Glycemic index and dietary fibre and the risk of type 2 diabetes. Diabetes Care, Nov. 27(11):2701–2706.

insulin secretion resulting in steadier blood sugar levels and a lower risk of diabetes.[17]

One of the theories put forward to explain why obesity and diabetes are so prevalent now is the "Thrifty Gene Hypothesis." Before the agricultural revolution there were times of feast and famine. People whose bodies had the capacity to put food into storage were more likely to survive times of crop failure and live until food was again available. Natural selection then ensured that these "thrifty genes" were passed on. Today, with highly processed food so readily available, this genetic advantage has turned into a disadvantage in that these individuals now store calories too quickly, leading to significant health problems. It is important to note, however, that when these high GI foods are left out of the diet, a healthy weight can be maintained.

**2. Eat fewer bad fats**. Good fats such as the omega-3 fatty acids discussed above reduce inflammation in the body by lowering hormone-like substances called prostaglandins. Bad—saturated—fats have the opposite effect, and therefore contribute to numerous illnesses including heart disease, stroke, Alzheimer's dementia and arthritis. Saturated fats are found in animal products such as meats, especially fatty meats, as well as cheese and other high fat dairy products. It is therefore prudent to reduce consumption of these foods.

Even worse are the plant oils that are synthetically

---

[17] Davis, M. S., et.al, 2004, More favorable dietary patterns are associated with lower glycemic load in older adults. *Journal of the American Dietetic Association*, Dec.104 (12):1828–1835.

hardened to prolong shelf life. Oils, that are liquid at room temperature, can become rancid over time. Through a process called hydrogenation, these oils can be turned solid thereby reducing the risk of spoilage. This process was first patented in 1902, and in 1911, Crisco became the first vegetable oil shortening made of hydrogenated cottonseed oil, revolutionizing the baking industry. Until recently, most commercially available baked goods contained hydrogenated or partially hydrogenated oils, also called vegetable oil shortening or trans fatty acids (TFAs). Although steps are being taken to reduce these fats, they are still abundant in homes, schools, restaurants, and hospitals.

Unfortunately, hydrogenated oils pose a major health risk. As the plant oil goes from the liquid to solid form it becomes saturated with hydrogen ions and therefore increases the risk of heart disease just like animals fats such as lard and butter do. Because this is an artificial food, however, our bodies have not developed the enzymes to break these fats down. Synthetically hydrogenated trans fatty acids (TFAs) are worse than the naturally occurring ones. TFAs inhibit the natural conversion of omega-3 FAs (short chain ALA to long chain EPA and DHA) that are critical for many aspects of good health. In addition, as these modified fats are incorporated into the tissues of our bodies, mainly the cell membranes and our brains, they literally alter their architecture and function in an adverse manner.

Industrially-produced trans fats are, calorie for calorie, the most harmful substance in our diet. As already discussed, there are many risk factors for ill health, with trans fats being just one of them. However, most of the foods we eat have some health benefits, even though excessive consumption is harmful. Trans fats, on the other hand, are completely devoid of nutritional value and toxic to our bodies; much like cigarette smoke[18].

TFAs are harder on the heart and arteries than are saturated fats. They increase total cholesterol, raise "bad" LDL (low density lipoprotein) cholesterol and lower "good" HDL (high density lipoprotein) cholesterol. Beyond that, TFAs have adverse effects on cell membranes and the immune system, cause inflammation of blood vessels, and promote cancer and aging. Trans fats have been linked to type 2 diabetes, adult and childhood obesity, sudden heart attack, and Alzheimer's disease. The effects of trans fats on human health are devastating.

Check labels carefully and eliminate all foods that contain hydrogenated oils. These include most crackers and other commercially baked goods, breakfast cereals, snack bars, and candy bars. Several countries such as Denmark, Germany, and Japan have banned or are in the process of banning TFAs. Several restaurant chains and food manufacturers have taken TFCs out of their products. A few US cities, including New York and Philadelphia, have banned trans fats in schools and restaurants. In September, 2009, British Columbia was the first province in Canada to restrict trans fats in restaurants, delis, bakeries, school cafeterias, and health-care institutions.

**3. Reduce consumption of animal products** (meats and dairy products), which are often too high in protein as well as

---

[18] Blatherwick, John, former Vancouver Chief Medical Health Officer, 2007, "Death By Trans Fats—It's time to ban from our diets something that, like tobacco, has absolutely no health benefits." Editorial: *The Vancouver Sun*, 30 May Page: A19. (In 2007 Health Canada promised to put strict limits on trans fats in food products. However, as of 2012, this had still not been accomplished.)

saturated fats. Animal proteins are harder to digest than vegetable proteins and contribute to numerous health problems. Red meat consumption has been shown to increase mortality from cardiovascular disease and cancer as well as total mortality[19]. It is also important to not add harmful fats to foods when preparing meals. This includes butter, lard, bacon, and cheese, and the fats that are used to pan fry or deep fry foods. Deep fryers in particular can contain harmful oils when used over and over again. The frying process also adds *acrylamide* and other potentially toxic substances. Acrylamides are naturally occurring substances that form when foods are cooked, baked, or roasted. They are found in breads, potato chips, rice, grilled meats, and many other foods. Acrylamides have been around for as long as foods have been heated but are of concern as high levels are associated with increased cancer rates in animals.

Grilling meats so that they are charred can result in the formation of heterocyclic amines (HCA), which are known to be carcinogenic. High protein diets also contribute to hypertension and therefore heart disease as well as kidney disease.

Consuming animal proteins, in particular grilled meats, as well as sugar, increases the formation of *Advanced*

---

[19] Pan A., et al., 2012, Red Meat Consumption and Mortality, and accompanying editorial: Ornish, D., Holy cow! What's good for you is good for the planet. For each additional daily serving of red meat, total mortality was increased by 12%, cardiovascular mortality by 16% and cancer mortality by 10%. Processed red meats (especially bacon and hot dogs) had a higher mortality rate than unprocessed meats (beef, pork, lamb). *Archives of Internal Medicine*, published online, March 12, 2012. www.archinternmed.com.

*Glycation End-products (AGEs)*. These are pro-inflammatory molecules that contribute to diabetic and age-related complications including cardiovascular disease, strokes, dementia, cataracts, asthma, and arthritis. A diet high is whole grains, nuts, vegetables, and fish reduces the formation of these harmful substances.

A diet high in animal products is not only unhealthy, but also not globally sustainable. It can take about as much water to produce one pound of beef as it does to have a seven minute shower every day for a year! Furthermore, the immense amount of arable land required to pasture livestock is depleting grasslands and rainforests, which contributes to global warming. The destruction of habitat has resulted in reduced biodiversity with the loss of countless species of birds and other creatures. In addition, the cruelty and suffering that animals are subjected to in factory farms simply cannot be condoned if one is eating with conscience. Hence, there are dramatic and far-reaching improvements in human and global health with a shift to a plant-based diet[20].

By fostering the habit of simultaneously consuming more of the unprocessed nutritious foods while systematically cutting out harmful foods, significant health improvements can result. In this way, an ideal diet can be more easily achieved and maintained.

---

[20] Author, John Robbins, (1987, Diet for a New America, and 2001, The Food Revolution, How Your Diet can Help Save Your Life and the World) has written clearly and eloquently about how meat production has a devastating global impact through the depletion of natural resources, and how high meat consumption has a negative effect on human health.

David was amazed at how much he had already gleaned from the booklet. He had previously paid scant attention to nutrition, other than to eat what he enjoyed when he was hungry. Who knew that what you ate had a direct influence on your health? Now that he had a framework to follow, he realized that it would not be difficult to make healthier food choices. He needed to get ready for his doctor's appointment but not before he had read another paragraph that caught his eye.

**One minute message**

Food choices have a remarkably *consistent* effect on health outcomes.

A diet that is high in whole grains, nuts, fruits, veggies, and high in OMEGA-3 fatty acids *reduces inflammation.* This lowers the risk of heart disease, stroke, cancer, arthritis, osteoporosis, dementia, and depression. It may even *slow the aging process.*

Losing weight is simple. It is not easy, but it is simple; one needs to create a caloric deficit. We understand financial deficits that occur when individuals or governments spend more money than they bring in. In the same way, if more calories are expended than are consumed, weight loss occurs. Quite simply, there are two variables that can be controlled that influence weight: caloric intake and energy expenditure. In addition, some people burn calories quicker than others because of differences in their metabolism. While thyroid disease and other medical conditions occasionally contribute to obesity and need to be ruled out, a major determinant of resting metabolic rate is lean body mass. Muscle burns approximately twenty-five times more energy than fat even at rest. This is why lean and muscular individuals literally lose weight while they sleep or lounge around a swimming pool. This is also why strength training, as well as aerobic conditioning, is critical to good health and maintenance of normal weight.

---

David arrived at the doctor's office fifteen minutes ahead of schedule and completed some registration forms. He was ushered into an examination room where he reflected for a few minutes on the wealth of knowledge he'd spent the day reading.

"Hi David, I'm Peter Osler," said the physician as the two men shook hands. David wondered when they had started letting children into medical school. Dr. Osler looked as if he did not need to shave yet, but David soon realized that his new doc was older and more experienced than he appeared. He had a fresh complexion, lean athletic build and was dressed in casual khaki pants and a white golf shirt.

Osler had moved to British Columbia from Saskatchewan as his wife, Madeline, was from Vancouver. They both preferred the climate on the West Coast. He had worked in several towns in BC in the last years, but had settled on the North Shore as it was close to skiing and mountain biking opportunities. He enjoyed what the province had to offer and made a point of doing a longer hike at least once a month.

Most of these were day trips to some of the local mountains, but his favourite had been a week on the West Coast Trail hiking through the ancient rain forests on the western coast of Vancouver Island. He had sailed to Desolation Sound with one of his colleagues and also loved exploring the coves and inlets along the shore by ocean kayak.

"Hi, I'm David Mackenzie. Thanks for seeing me on such short notice. I guess you know that I had a car accident and a bit of a heart attack last week?"

"Yes, I got that information, but don't know much else about you. Today, I'd like to get some history, and then we'll book you for a thorough physical. By that time I hope your hospital records will have arrived, and then we'll work together to reduce your risk of another heart attack."

Dr. Osler's professional but engaging manner put David at ease and increased his level of confidence in the younger man. Osler explored David's past medical history, family history, social history, and habits to determine his cardiac risk. David was a bit surprised when Osler asked him if he had many friends and what he did in his spare time.

"Okay, David … you have just been given a wake-up call. You are a forty-two-year-old man who has survived his first heart attack, and it is now largely up to you whether you can extend your own warranty, or whether you want to take your chances on surviving a second heart attack. I'm a little worried that if you keep doing what you have being doing up until now, you may suffer another heart attack. I'd like to help you make some changes that will improve your odds."

"It seems to me," Dr. Osler continued, "that young people can often get away with sleepless nights, too much partying with excessive alcohol consumption, smoking, and eating whatever they please. I don't condone a reckless lifestyle at all, but young people can tolerate a lot, as their bodies are remarkably forgiving and heal quickly. Unfortunately, for some of them, their poor judgment leads to sexually transmitted diseases, substance abuse and addiction, or serious injury or even death following a motor vehicle accident."

"Eventually, however, everyone pays a price. Somewhere around age forty the warranty expires, and it's time to make wise choices or face the consequences. I can help regulate your medications, and believe me, it is critical that you take them, but there are other significant factors that are going to determine the quality and quantity of your remaining years."

"Do you mean my diet? I've been giving that some thought actually, and I'm ready to make some changes. Maybe you could help me with that area," replied David.

"Yes, I do mean your diet; however, I prefer to call it nutrition, as diet is a four-letter word that sounds too temporary. Indeed, I would be happy to help you in that regard. Most of us eat too much, and many of us eat way too much. Over-nutrition, which leads to obesity, is now a larger problem globally than malnutrition. But there is much more to a healthy lifestyle than what you put in your mouth. You are going to have to start on a regular exercise program, and also closely examine your life to determine your stressors and how you can lessen their impact on your physical and mental well-being."

"Exercise program? I'm not sure how I would fit it in. I'm pretty busy with work, and I try to be involved in my kids' lives as well."

"What would you find easier to fit into your busy lifestyle—thirty minutes of exercise a day or being dead twenty-four hours a day?" quipped Osler.

"Seriously, a brisk fifteen-minute walk each day, rain or shine, is a great start, although, it would be ideal to see a trainer and start on a regular program. Did they mention cardiac rehab at St. Luke's?" queried the physician.

David remembered Dr. Schreiber saying something about a rehab program, and felt confident that his family doctor was up to speed with current recommendations. Osler advised him that he could attend the supervised exercise classes through the local YMCA. There is also the opportunity to register with the Centre for Active Living, an innovative concept in healthcare. It is a facility built by our Hospital and Community Health Foundation in which an integrated team of care providers help patients to take control of chronic health conditions through education, nutrition, and exercise.

David thanked Dr. Osler for his time and on his way out scheduled an appointment for his physical exam for the following week. Dr. Osler had also reminded him to have a dental check-up and an eye exam as part of his comprehensive health assessment.

Peter Osler took a moment to think about his new patient. He often attended patients who had serious and chronic health conditions for which they alone were responsible. Typically, his patients were not even aware nor did they care how their lifestyle choices were affecting their health. Osler loved the work that he did; he felt that it was a privilege to help his patients through illnesses and life transitions. He regretted that he often felt rushed and that he was not able to inspire more of his patients to make appropriate lifestyle changes. He saw many of them heading down a destructive road, yet felt powerless and frustrated at times that he was not able to intervene more meaningfully within the context of the limited office visit.

Dr. Osler hoped that David would have the courage to make the necessary changes in order to improve his chances of living as full a life as possible. After a major illness, many of his patients vowed to make significant and permanent changes, but unfortunately their motivation was not often sustained. Peter Osler hoped that he could be a catalyst for change in David Mackenzie's case. He also recognized that ultimately it would be up to David himself to do the hard work. He knew that "you can lead a horse to water …"

*Every system is perfectly designed to get the results it achieves.*

**Donald Berwick**
(1946–), American health administrator

# CHAPTER 3

*"All the flowers of all the tomorrows are in the seeds of today and yesterday"*

**Chinese proverb**

The Kitsilano Orcas had not won a game all season. David had agreed to be the assistant coach for Adam's Under-9 soccer team so that Adam could play on the same team as his best buddy, Mathias, whose father was the coach. Between his hectic work schedule and the separation from Jessica, however, David rarely made it to any of the games, much less the practices. Today was different. He surprised the team by showing up for practice with some new drills he had gotten from a client who had once coached for the Vancouver Whitecaps. He had picked up some chocolate glazed doughnuts for the kids as a treat for having worked hard in their practice.

Jessica picked Adam up after the practice and immediately spied the now-empty doughnut box. "When are you going to stop feeding the kids that toxic junk-food?" she asked abruptly.

"Uh, nice to see you too, dear, yes, I'm feeling much better, thanks," he replied.

David asked if he could come over for supper, but Jessica said she would prefer another time. The kids had to do homework and practise piano, and she needed to prepare her lesson plan for the next day. Chastened, David made his way to Yaletown, let himself into his lonely apartment and after wandering aimlessly around for a few minutes, he picked up his book again. It was compelling reading for a man who'd suffered a heart attack in the prime of his life. For the second time in as many days he wondered whether it was merely coincidence that he had been the one to find it in the cab on his way home from the hospital. Or was it serendipity?

*When you get older it is not so important **what** you do—just **that** you do.*

**Erhardt Spangehl (1924–)**

## HABIT TWO: EXERCISE

Our bodies, like those of other animals, are designed to be active. Early human beings roamed in social groups for most of the day, gathering food, hunting, playing, and reproducing. Although our challenges in the twenty-first century are different, we are still hardwired from those days as predators, and we must still respect and understand that fundamental blueprint.

Living creatures are continuously replacing and renewing cells and tissues that have been injured, died, or have passed their "best before date." Recall that in Habit One: Diet, the importance of selecting high quality building materials was recommended for this reason. Cellular death—or apoptosis—followed by cellular renewal is a process that persists from infancy to our death. As we get older, the renewal and healing process can slow down. However, we can influence whether our bodies are tilted more to the growth and renewal side or to the death and decay side. The signal that stimulates growth—of bone, muscle, connective tissue, blood vessels, and even brain cells—is *exercise!* Exercise is literally the Fountain of Youth for the body and the brain. It improves blood flow to the brain, and therefore, concentration and mood. The more active we are, the more our tissues get stressed and damaged and then renew and grow to improve strength and function. Stagnation, on the other hand, leads to loss of function, cellular decay, and eventually, illness and death.

Our bodies and brains crave this activity and are therefore at odds with the reality that we now spend most of our days sitting in front of computer screens, commuting to work, and largely engaging in sedentary pursuits. We do these things because we need to in order to find food, shelter, and provide for our families in our civilization. However, because our bodies so require movement, it is critical that we make the time to exercise every day. Brisk walks are a good start and when done regularly contribute to good health. However, in order to signal our bodies to grow and renew, it is necessary to stress the body by participating in vigorous aerobic, resistance, and flexibility training at least three to four times a week.

**One minute message**

*Exercise* signals growth and *renewal* in the body, versus cellular death and *decay*.

To obtain the multiple and dramatic benefits from exercise, and to cut the risk of dying of a heart attack in half, you need to be moderately active for at least an hour each day, and engage in *vigorous* exercise for at least thirty minutes three to four times per week.

This should include: *cardiovascular fitness, weight training*, as well as *flexibility* and *balance* exercises.

"Maintaining ideal body weight is important in preventing decline in overall health and physical functioning. However, regular exercise can reduce the risk of health decline even among individuals who cannot achieve ideal weight[21]. In other words, you are better off being fat and fit rather than thin and out of shape.

Motivation comes in many forms. In order to get the most benefit from exercising and to reduce the risk of injury it is advisable to work with a trainer to create a program that combines stretching, strengthening, and cardiovascular fitness. Group classes, boot camps, or working with a training partner all provide enjoyment and camaraderie. Physical fitness includes: resistance training to improve strength, power, and muscle endurance; aerobic conditioning to improve cardiovascular endurance; as well as exercises to improve flexibility, balance, and coordination.

*Aerobic* activities refer to those that burn oxygen. Any activity that uses large muscle groups, is rhythmic in nature, and can be sustained for long periods of time, can be defined as an aerobic exercise. It results in a moderate increase not only in heart rate but also in breathing rate. Aerobic exercises condition the heart, lungs, and circulatory system by causing them to work harder than when at rest. Common examples include brisk walking, hiking, jogging/running, swimming, rowing, stair climbing, bicycling, cross-country skiing, and aerobics

---

[21] He, X.Z., Baker, D.W., 2004, Body Mass Index, Physical Activity, and the Risk of Decline in Overall Health and Physical Functioning in Late Middle Age, *American Journal of Public Health*, September, 94, No. 9, 1567–1573.

classes. The key is doing these exercises for long periods of time at sub-maximal levels wherein you can still carry on a conversation.

Aerobic exercises involve back and forth movement of large muscle groups to strengthen the cardiovascular system. When you exercise, the muscles demand more oxygen-rich blood and give off more carbon dioxide and other waste. This makes your heart beat faster to keep up and opens up the blood vessels as well.

When you follow a program of regular aerobic exercise, over time your heart and blood vessels grow stronger and can meet the muscles' demands without as much effort. With improved cardiovascular fitness the resting heart rate will decline, and the time it takes the heart rate to return to normal after exercise will improve as well. Both men and women benefit equally from improved cardiovascular fitness. Check with your doctor first if you have a chronic condition or are overweight, are a smoker, or are middle aged or older and have never exercised.

**How to achieve aerobic fitness**

To strengthen your heart, you should do aerobic exercise intensely enough to reach your target heart rate. This is 60–80 percent of your maximum heart rate, which can be estimated by subtracting your age from 220. (For example, if you're fifty years old, your maximum heart rate is 170 and your target heart rate is 102–136; at sixty, your maximum heart rate is 160 and your target heart rate is 96–128.) This estimate is a safe place to start an exercise program and may suffice for most people. If you are serious about more intense training, talk to your doctor about getting a stress test to determine your true maximum heart rate so you can calculate your specific target heart rate more precisely.

In order to accurately check your heart rate, it is essential to invest in a heart rate monitor. These are not expensive, are readily available, and will definitely help you to improve your level of fitness. Next, calculate your maximum heart rate and memorize your target range.

Aerobic conditioning involves two stages. The first and most important is doing slow and steady activities at the lower end of the target range (60–65 percent of maximum) for long periods of time of time—such as hiking or cycling for one to two hours. When a good aerobic base has been established in this manner, activity levels should be increased to get into the higher end of the target heart rate (75–80 percent of maximum). This includes faster jogging, uphill climbs when hiking or cycling, swimming, rowing, or any other moderately intense activity. The duration of this more challenging sustained activity level should be gradually increased to a period of thirty minutes or longer while maintaining approximately 75–80 percent of your maximum heart rate.

Think of *aerobic activity* as being *long in duration yet moderate and sustainable in intensity*. These activities require oxygen to make the energy needed for prolonged exercise and improve your cardiovascular system. Aerobic activities use mainly the "slow twitch" muscle fibres which allow slow and steady muscle contractions and improve *endurance*.

*Anaerobic activity*, on the other hand, is *short in duration and high in intensity*. Anaerobic activities include: weight lifting, racquetball, downhill skiing, sprinting, basketball, soccer, football, and others. Most team sports have an aerobic as well as anaerobic component. Anaerobic activities use predominantly the "fast twitch" muscle fibres, which are needed for strength and power.

When doing aerobic exercises ("with air or oxygen") you should be able to carry on a short conversation. If you are gasping for air while talking, you are probably working anaerobically. When you work anaerobically, you will tire faster and are more likely to experience sore muscles after exercise is over. With more conditioning, aerobic capacity improves and you should be able to carry on the exercises with less effort and breathlessness.

The term *anaerobic* means *without air* or *without oxygen*. Anaerobic exercise uses muscles at high intensity and a high rate of work for a short period of time. Anaerobic exercise helps us increase our muscle strength and prepare us for quick bursts of power and speed. During intense anaerobic activities, near maximal heart rate (90–100 percent) is achieved.

Think of the energy output of a cornered animal fighting for its life. This short and intense activity is anaerobic exercise. Pushing our heart rate into this high performance range should only be done when a good aerobic base has been built by doing the slow and steady aerobic training for hours at a time. Cardiovascular fitness can be achieved by initially working at 60 percent of your maximum heart rate, then up to 80 percent, and finally, doing intervals where the heart rate is pushed to near maximum for short periods of time.

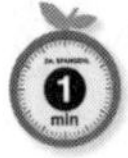

**One minute message**

To increase cardiovascular fitness, get a heart rate monitor and calculate your maximum heart rate by subtracting your age from 220.

1. Build an aerobic base by exercising at 60-65 percent of maximum. Continue training until you can sustain this heart rate for one hour.
2. Increase aerobic capacity by exercising at 75-80 percent of maximum until you can sustain this activity for thirty minutes.
3. Push your heart rate to 95-100 percent for short intervals to build anaerobic capacity.
4. Check how quickly your heart rate returns to normal after you finish exercising.

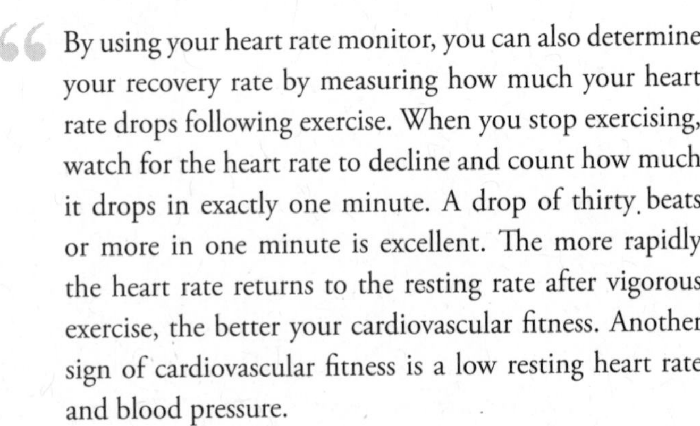

“By using your heart rate monitor, you can also determine your recovery rate by measuring how much your heart rate drops following exercise. When you stop exercising, watch for the heart rate to decline and count how much it drops in exactly one minute. A drop of thirty beats or more in one minute is excellent. The more rapidly the heart rate returns to the resting rate after vigorous exercise, the better your cardiovascular fitness. Another sign of cardiovascular fitness is a low resting heart rate and blood pressure.

Anaerobic exercises cannot last long because oxygen is not used for energy and a by-product, called lactic acid, is produced. *Lactic acid* contributes to muscle fatigue and must be burned up by the body during a recovery period before another anaerobic bout of exercise can be attempted. The recovery period also allows the muscles to use oxygen to replenish the energy used during the high-intensity exercise. The build-up of lactic acid is what makes muscles sore the day after exercising hard.

Both aerobic and anaerobic exercises are needed for the development of physical fitness. Check with your healthcare provider before you start an exercise program. Choose activities that you enjoy, and that are readily accessible as you will want to do them a lot.

As you first start to exercise—whether you are walking, running or lifting—your muscles will immediately require energy to allow them to work. For the first three minutes or so your muscles will burn a fuel called glycogen. This is a special sugar which is stored in the muscles for a quick infusion of energy. Some glycogen is always stored within your muscle tissues. During this period fat is not burned and oxygen is not used. So this is anaerobic metabolism. Often during the first few minutes of strenuous activity, especially during anaerobic metabolism, you may experience burning in muscles of your arms, legs, or back. This sensation is due to the creation of lactic acid which occurs when glycogen is burned and will soon go away.

As you exercise more than three minutes or so you will eventually burn up all of the glycogen stored within the muscles, and your muscles will move into aerobic metabolism. When this occurs, lactic acid production is stopped. At this time, glycogen, which is stored in the liver, is now being burned in the presence of oxygen, which is brought to the muscles by way of the blood stream. As long as you breathe correctly you will bring oxygen to the muscles and this process will continue.

Oxygen is essential to the muscle's ability to function correctly. With adequate oxygen the muscles can extract all the energy they need from blood sugar. During the period you exercise, the liver and muscles will release their stored carbohydrates to be used as energy by the muscles, thereby allowing you to keep on exercising.

Once all of the stored glycogen is used up—usually after about twenty minutes—the body will start burning its fat stores to produce blood sugar and ultimately glycogen. This is why you need to do sustained aerobic activities to burn fat. The longer you exercise the more fat is burned. Fat—that is stored body fat and not dietary fat—can now be used virtually indefinitely to produce energy to support your exercise program. While you are walking, you do not directly burn fat, but once you stop walking the glycogen that has been burned up must be replaced. This can only happen by what you eat and by the liver drawing fat from the body's fat tissues. If you are on a limited caloric intake then the food you ingest will be used basically for feeding your brain, and fat stores will have to be drawn upon to replace the glycogen used up while exercising.

Studies show that *fat-burning* may last for anywhere from six to twenty-four hours after exercise. You do not have to work out intensely or exert great effort when you exercise. The percentage of energy contributed from burning fat decreases as you increase the intensity of your exercise program. Prolonged mild to moderate aerobic exercise on a regular basis is an achievable goal worth striving for.

**Benefits of Regular Exercise:**

1. Exercise builds muscle mass. Larger muscles burn more calories than smaller muscles. Overdoing cardiovascular exercises can increase hunger and will not increase muscle mass which is needed to burn calories even at rest. For this reason it is important to include strength training in a weight loss program[22]. It also means that with larger muscles you can eat more without gaining weight.

2. Moderate exercise can decrease your appetite. Studies have shown us that light exercise increases appetite while heavy exercise decreases appetite initially, but within a short time appetite will increase. Moderate activity, on the other hand, lowers appetite and decreases your desire to eat.

3. Exercise helps to reduce stress and depression, both of which are common causes of overeating. While exercising regularly for extended periods of time, endorphins are released, which make you feel better. These

---

[22] Vincent, K.R., et. al., 2002, Improved cardiorespiratory endurance following 6 months of resistance exercise in elderly men and women. *Archives of Internal Medicine*, 162:673–678.

natural opioid chemicals diminish depression and relieve stress. This accounts for the "runner's high" that some athletes experience. In addition, levels of the neurotransmitters serotonin and dopamine are elevated, which contribute to the feeling of accomplishment and satisfaction that often occur after a vigorous workout. (Many anti-depressant medications increase the levels of these same neurotransmitters.) As circulation to the brain improves with exercise, more blood and therefore oxygen and nutrients can be used, resulting in improved mood, concentration, and cognitive function.

4. Physical exercise is one of the few techniques shown to increase the creation and connections of new neurons in the brain. Regular walking for at least an hour a day, along with a Mediterranean diet and learning new information are the most effective strategies for reducing the risk of dementia.

5. Exercise reduces your risk of heart disease by improving cardiovascular fitness and endurance. By stressing the heart, the cardiac arteries are widened and small new blood vessels may form to better deliver oxygen to the exercising muscle. Exercise has been shown to cut the risk of dying from a heart attack by 50 percent.

6. During exercise, systolic blood pressure (BP) rises (as a result of increased heart rate and cardiac output) and diastolic BP drops (because of blood vessels dilating and thus reducing peripheral resistance). With

regular exercise, resting blood pressure and heart rate are reduced. Again, this effect is augmented when an individual eats a diet low in animal protein, fat, and salt, and high in complex carbohydrates, rich in fibre, potassium, and magnesium.

> Contrary to previous belief, adults can form new brain cells; this is called neurogensis. Exercise, some anti-depressant medications, and surprisingly, electro-convulsive therapy are the strongest stimuli for the formation of new brain cells. Physical exercise, cognitive exercises, happiness, as well as new challenges and life experiences also improve neuroplasticity—the ability of existing brain tissue to develop new functions. An old dog can learn new tricks!
>
> As the prevalence of dementia is projected to rise dramatically over the next decades, and since medications improve symptoms only modestly, risk factor modification remains the cornerstone of dementia prevention. This includes management of vascular risk factors—especially hypertension and diabetes, cognitive activities, physical exercise, recognition and treatment of depression, and a diet, rich in antioxidants and polyunsaturated fatty acids.[23]

7. Exercise increases HDL-cholesterol (the "good" cholesterol) and diminishes LDL-cholesterol (the "bad" cholesterol).

8. Exercise reduces the risk of diabetes by increasing the

---

[23] Middleton, L, et. al., 2009, Promising Strategies for the Prevention of Dementia, *Archives of Neurology*, October, 66(10): 1210-1215.

use of sugar in a healthy and productive way. It also helps because fat is lost and muscle mass is increased.

9. Regular exercise improves heart muscle efficiency. With exercise, the heart muscle becomes stronger, pumps better, and more blood is pumped with each contraction. This means the heart does not have to work as hard to circulate the blood.

10. As important as exercise is to strengthening the heart, it is also the key to maintaining soft and flexible arteries that are less likely to clog up with plaque. Exercise improves circulation to the coronary arteries (as well as the rest of the body) as the increased cardiac output and reduced peripheral resistance increase flow through vessels and stimulate *angioneogenesis*—the formation of new arteries (i.e. the stimulatory effects of vigorous exercise result in a mini-bypass effect through areas that do not receive enough oxygen.)

11. Regular exercise will decrease the risk of osteoporosis in men and women. Exercise strengthens bones, making them less likely to break.

12. Exercise can help you to sleep better.

13. Regular exercise helps to keep the bowels moving on a regular basis.

14. Exercise will also improve the function of weight-bearing joints as it massages the cartilages and the

shock-absorbing menisci in the knees to improve the flow of nutrients to these structures.

15. Exercise improves the function of the immune system. While we have a fixed number of chromosomes in each cell, specific genes that improve cellular and immune function can be expressed through exercise. Therefore, regular exercise can help to decrease the risk of many different illnesses. However, over exercising can lead to injuries and in some cases even weaken the immune system, so it is important to remember the maxim "everything in moderation."

16. With regular moderate exercise, you not only feel better but also look better, thus stimulating self-image and self-esteem.

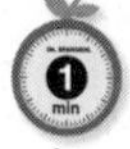

**One minute message**

If you do not have time for regular exercise, remember that doing something is better than doing *nothing*.

Stand on one foot when tying your shoe laces, take the stairs, sit on an exercise ball at your desk or when watching a movie, or take a dog for a walk.

Many people are simply not able to get to a gym or commit to a regular fitness program. Others feel that they work hard enough physically, and that the last thing they need is to exercise. In fact, hard manual labour is like performing a sport, and to reduce injury it is even more important to be fit, strong, and flexible. Furthermore, the benefits of exercise are more than just the cardiovascular conditioning and strengthening achieved. Making time for *deliberate exercise* reinforces the importance of spending time for ourselves. Studies have shown that exercising in our leisure time has more benefits than physically demanding work. This may be because the exercise is done in a stress-free setting and not because the boss is putting us under pressure to produce.[24]

Far from being selfish, nurturing ourselves through a healthy diet, regular exercise, holidays, and recreation, makes us more productive in the work we do, and more effective in our relationships with others.

Making a decision to increase one's level of fitness and therefore improve one's general health can begin with small, easy steps that do not require a significant time commitment. A good place to start is with the exercises that follow.

**Better than Nothing exercises** are spending a small amount of time getting some deliberate exercise, either cardiovascular (eg. doing jumping jacks or skipping rope for three minutes) or strengthening ("Give me twenty push-ups!"). A good start to any exercise program is

---

[24] Nordstrom, C. K.., et. al., 2003, Leisure time physical activity and early atherosclerosis: the Los Angeles Atherosclerosis Study. *American Journal of Medicine*, Jul; 115(1): 19–25.

to take a walk. This can be as little as ten minutes in the morning before work, or a short walk on a coffee break or at lunchtime. The benefits far exceed the small amount of time spent.

**Incidental exercises** are "freebies." They involve the same amount of time doing what one would normally do, but doing it in a way that simultaneously improves your strength and fitness. Sit on an exercise ball while watching a movie or while working at your desk or while you are eating. To improve balance and core muscle strength, put on and tie your shoes while standing, lifting your feet alternately. Brush your teeth while standing on one leg with your eyes closed. Stretch while watching TV, or during a car or plane trip.

You don't need to work out frantically every day to improve your health and prevent chronic disease. Optimal exercise to improve cardiovascular fitness, strength, flexibility and endurance requires at least sixty to ninety minutes a day. Yet, many experts agree that thirty minutes of moderate physical activity on most days of the week will improve your cardiovascular fitness, as well as reduce the risk of developing many degenerative diseases. Health benefits can be derived by taking small periods of exercise frequently; three ten-minute walks after meals give the same benefit as one thirty-minute walk.

Bear in mind that staying in "cruise control" will not improve health and reduce the effects of aging. A daily effort to push one's boundaries and comfort zone will help you to reap the numerous benefits of regular exercise.

"*Incidental exercises* involve the same amount of time doing what one would normally do, but doing it in a way that simultaneously improves your strength and fitness."

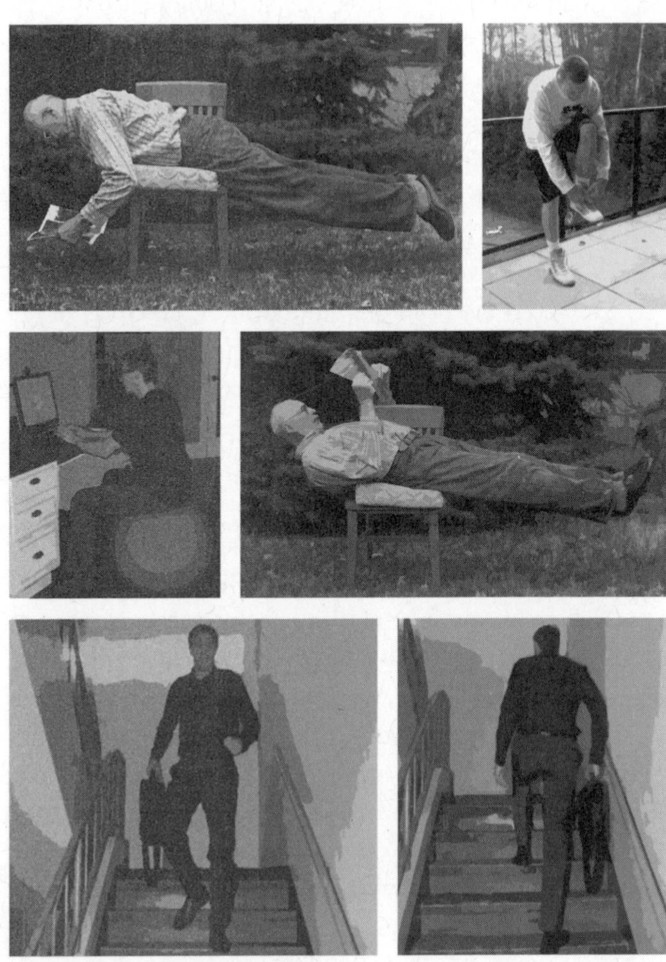

"Try some of these ideas to increase the amount of physical activity you get each day.

- Take the stairs instead of the elevator at work. Walking up five flights of stairs at a moderate pace will elevate the heart rate and burn ten to twenty calories, depending on your weight. (Calories Burned Estimators available on-line allow you to calculate the number of calories burned doing everyday activities.)
- Park the car at the far end of the parking lot and walk to your destination.
- Walk or cycle in your local communities as you do your errands. No need to burn fossil fuels when we can burn our own fuel.
- Walk the dog around the soccer field while attending your child's sports practice. (If you do not have a dog—borrow one; friends are always happy to have their dogs walked!)
- Suck in your stomach (pull your belly button towards your spine and upwards) while driving the car or working at the computer or when sitting and waiting. Engaging your core muscles in this way before bending and lifting will also reduce back pains.
- Organize a fitness challenge in your workplace.
- Take dancing lessons.

**Yoga** reduces anxiety, stress and pain and increases flexibility, strength, balance and well-being. Practicing yoga has been shown to be helpful in treating a multitude of medical conditions including hypertension, headaches, fibromyalgia, asthma, chronic lung disease, heart and circulatory disease, diabetes, osteoporosis, arthritis, multiple sclerosis, infertility and depression. Yoga can instil a sense of calm by decreasing blood pressure, heart rate, and stress hormones, through the production of three compounds that promote relaxation.

The runner's high and increasing neurotransmitter levels have been mentioned as an effect of aerobic exercise. Yoga has also been shown to result in a natural high by boosting blood levels of serotonin, dopamine, and endorphins—three natural "feel-good" substances. *Serotonin* is a neurotransmitter that makes you feel cheerful and content. *Dopamine* is a brain chemical closely tied to the pleasure centers of the brain. It is a satisfaction peptide that is elevated when you feel a sense of accomplishment or get positive feedback. And *endorphins* are the opiate-like compounds that produce a sense of well-being.

You don't need to be an expert to reap the benefits from yoga—just trying beginner poses will result in health improvements. Yoga makes you fitter by incorporating dynamic and symmetrical stretches.

Muscles aren't static tissues; they need to move, expand, and contract. The more flexible they are, the better range of motion you will enjoy, and the less tension you'll put on your joints as you pursue normal activities. Yoga increases your overall strength without using weights. The poses engage your muscles in lifting and holding your body weight. This counts as resistance training.

Doing the *Sun Salutation* every day works most of your muscle groups in one flowing routine.

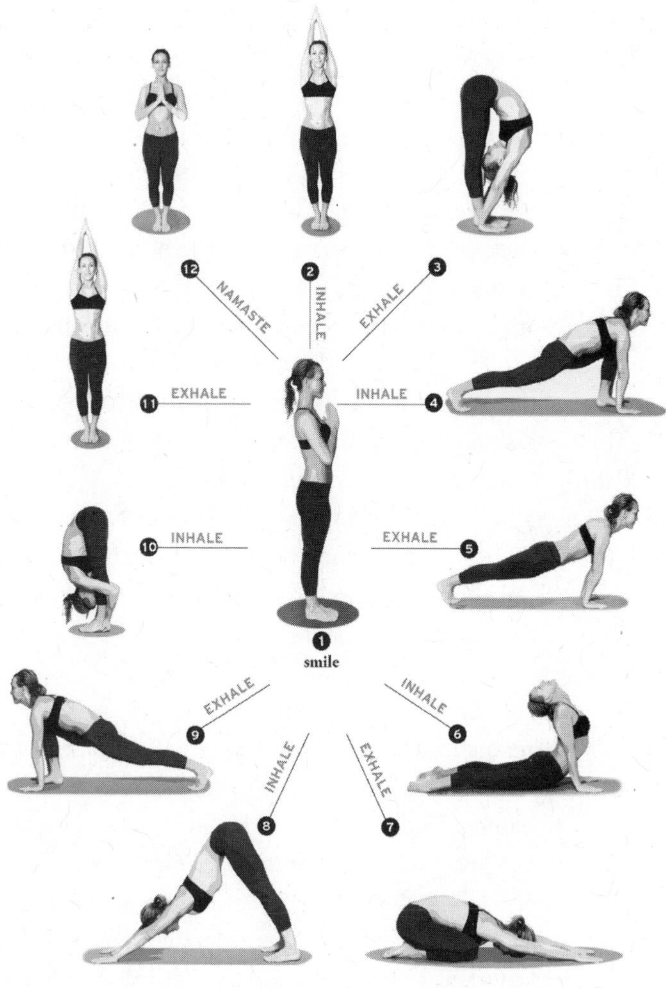

Start the sequence by standing comfortably, with feet together, and hands held in prayer. Keep your hands together as you extend them above your head and stretch backwards. Bend forwards and touch the floor. Stretch your right leg out behind you and keep your left leg at 90 degrees (Lunge). Stretch both legs behind you in a Plank. Lay on your abdomen with your palms flat on the ground while lifting your head and shoulders up (Upward Dog). Optional: open your mouth as widely as possible, stick out your tongue and roar! (Lion Pose). Keep your hands where they are and bend your knees to tuck your buttocks onto your heels (Child's Pose). Lift your buttocks in the air with your arms and legs straight (Downward Dog). Keep the left leg stretched out behind you and bend your right leg 90 degrees. Stand up while keeping your hands on the floor. Stand up fully with hands extended into a backbend. End as you started, standing comfortably, feet together, hands in prayer, and smiling.

Remember, the full benefits from yoga are obtained by trying your best. It is not necessary to do the postures perfectly. It's all about going as far as you can in each pose and continuing your practice.

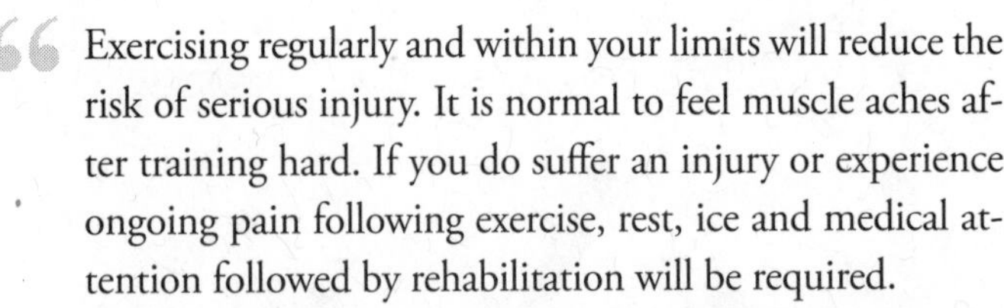

" Exercising regularly and within your limits will reduce the risk of serious injury. It is normal to feel muscle aches after training hard. If you do suffer an injury or experience ongoing pain following exercise, rest, ice and medical attention followed by rehabilitation will be required.

While regular exercise is important and hard training is critical to peak performances in sport, it is important to avoid overtraining, which increases the risk of injury. A wise coach and a smart athlete both realize that it takes a long time to come back after a serious injury, so appropriate times of rest and recovery are necessary in any training program to avoid the hazards of overdoing a good thing. By exercising consistently and avoiding injury you can stay active and fit well into your senior years.

..................................................................................

David spent much of the week watching TV, reading, and resting. Unaccustomed to spending so much time in his apartment, he made a concerted effort to clean and organize it. He had decided to slowly start his own exercise routine, and began each day with a walk after breakfast. One day he walked half an hour to the Vancouver Public Library, and on the spur of the moment, registered for a library card, something he had not had in his possession since childhood. He made his way to the "Diet and Exercise" section and picked out several books, some of which seemed to recommend completely opposite approaches.

There was a message on his answering machine when he arrived home. Dr. Osler's office had called to advise that his appointment was going to be two hours later than scheduled. The doctor had delivered a baby that morning so some of his appointments needed to be moved. The delay gave David time to do a load of laundry, snack on some fruit and start reading his new finds before catching a cab to Dr. Osler's office.

..................................................................................

David soon realized that this was not going to be an in-and-out appointment at a walk-in clinic. An assistant weighed and measured him and checked both his blood pressure and vision. He was then asked to strip to his shorts and wait for the doctor. When Osler arrived he calculated David's Body Mass Index (BMI). This is a height to weight measurement easily calculated and recorded on the Electronic Medical Record. David's BMI was 29 kg/m$^2$, at the high end of the "overweight" range; 30 or greater is considered "obese."

"What should I be aiming for?" asked David with a hint of anxiety.

"The norm for men is 20–25," replied Osler. "Bear in mind that for muscular men BMI is not as predictive of cardiac risk as abdominal circumference. For example, Wayne Gretzky had a BMI of 29 when he played hockey for the Edmonton Oilers, but he had a slim waist and was certainly fit and not overweight."

> An abdominal circumference of greater than 94 cm (37") in men and 80 cm (32") in women is associated with a higher risk of heart disease. These numbers apply to Caucasians. For Asian populations (Chinese, Japanese, and South Asians) the risk of heart disease increases with an abdominal girth of greater than 88 cm (35") for men and 80 cm (32") for women. Until specific data for African Americans is available, it is assumed that the risk is similar to populations of European ancestry.[25]

---

[25] Genest, Jacques MD, et al., Oct. 2009, "Canadian Guidelines for the diagnosis and treatment of dyslipidemia and prevention of cardiovascular disease in the adult, 2009 recommendations". *Canadian Journal of Cardiology*, Vol. 25 No 10. These guidelines were published by the Canadian Cardiovascular Society to bring North American populations in closer alignment with European recommendations.

David's girth—or waist circumference—was 112 cm. "I knew I was a bit flabby around the middle but had no idea that I am nearly 'obese' and that a single measurement can show that I'm at high risk for cardiac disease," said David quietly. "This is a real eye-opener."

David's blood pressure was 146/88 mm Hg. Osler checked the measurement again in both arms and the upper number was consistently over 140. "Hmmm … that's higher than it should be," said the doctor. "Normal BP is around 120/80 mm Hg. Do you want me to explain it further?"

David nodded assent.

"The upper number is the systolic BP which is the pressure when the heart is contracting, and the lower number is the diastolic pressure, which is when the heart is in relaxation and filling with blood again. High blood pressure—or *hypertension*—is defined as either systolic BP greater than 140 or diastolic pressure over 90 mm Hg," said Osler. "I know it's a lot to take in, but, believe me, blood pressure is a key determinant of your health."

Dr. Osler asked David if he would measure his blood pressure several times in a pharmacy and to bring those readings to his next appointment. "Then we will measure your blood pressure again here to confirm the diagnosis," he added.

David looked at the doctor with concern. It was becoming obvious that his heart attack was going to precipitate a new chapter in his adult life.

"There are many medications that we use to control blood pressure," began Osler. "Although you may need one or more in the future, I would like you to start treating your blood pressure with some dietary and lifestyle changes."

The Seventh report of the Joint National Committee on the Prevention, Detection, Evaluation and Treatment of High Blood Pressure recommends that lifestyle modifications should be the initial treatment strategy for lowering BP. This includes weight reduction, physical activity, sodium restriction, moderation of alcohol intake and the DASH diet (JNC-7, NIH publication, 2004).

The original DASH Study (1993–1997) found that participants on the low fat, high fibre diet, high in fruits and vegetables and low-fat dairy products, in particular with sodium restriction, had a significant reduction in BP. While this was demonstrated in short term feeding studies it had not been shown in free-living individuals. The ENCORE Study looked at the DASH diet alone and in combination with supervised exercise and weight loss and found that the combination resulted in significantly reduced BP and risk of heart disease[26].

"To lower blood pressure without medications I often recommend three strategies and find that when these are applied conscientiously, they are about as effective as using two pills to control hypertension. The first is *diet.* There is an evidence-based diet called DASH—Dietary Approaches to Stop Hypertension. The DASH study found that people who eat lots of fruits and veggies, whole grains, and low fat dairy products, and cut back saturated fats and salt had lower BP than control subjects. When the DASH diet was

---

[26] Blumenthal James et.al., 2010, The ENCORE Study looked at Effects of the DASH Diet Alone and in Combination with Exercise and Weight Loss on Blood Pressure and Cardiovascular Biomarkers in Men and Women with High Blood Pressure, *Archives of Internal Medicine* Vol. 170 (No. 2) 126–135, Jan 25. This trial demonstrated that the DASH diet with a 500 calorie energy deficit to result in approximately 1 pound of wt. loss per week along with 3 sessions of supervised exercise a week resulted in a significantly reduced BP (average 16/10 mmHg) as well as lower cardiovascular risk markers compared to DASH alone or controls.

combined with weight loss and exercise, participants also enjoyed a lower risk of stroke and heart disease. So look up the DASH diet on the Internet and follow it. In a few weeks we can do a 24-hour urine collection and determine how much sodium and potassium you are excreting in a day; this will allow us to determine whether your diet is low enough in salt and high enough in potassium. While DASH was developed to lower blood pressure, there is emerging evidence that it can help control cholesterol levels and heart disease risk as well."

"The second strategy is *exercise.* I can't emphasize enough the importance of regular vigorous exercise on health, fitness, and longevity," Dr. Osler continued. "The more you exercise, the more you will maintain your body functions as you age. It's the old "use it or lose it" principle that applies here. It is important to be active for about sixty to ninety minutes a day. Even if you have a physical job, it is still important to get about thirty minutes of intentional exercise a day to elevate the heart rate. For those of us with fairly sedentary jobs, we need to get at least an hour a day of vigorous movement such as brisk walking, cycling, swimming, gardening, dancing, or whatever you prefer. In addition, we need to do some weight training to maintain muscle mass and bone density, and regular stretching to maintain flexibility and reduce risk of injury."

"I've got a long way to go," muttered David.

"And you're not alone," replied Osler. "Inactivity quickly leads to muscle loss and reduced functional capacity. In fact, for each day a hospital patient is on bed rest, it takes at least three days to return to baseline. So if someone has an injury or illness that lands them in hospital for even two weeks—it takes at least six weeks to restore muscle strength. This is why it is so important to stay active throughout our adult and senior years."

"I tell all my retired patients to do what my dad does. He says that his "job" is to walk from nine in the morning until noon, Monday through Friday—rain or snow or shine. He does not always enjoy it or want to go—but then he did not always enjoy going to work either. He is quite stubborn, so he goes without fail. He packs water, an apple and a granola bar, then walks for ninety minutes, sits down and has his snack and then walks ninety minutes home again. He has a few destinations that he can reach right from his house, and on other days he drives to a trail head for variety. That still gives him plenty of time to do volunteer work, take continuing education courses and go travelling with my mom. The walking keeps the heart, lungs, and muscles toned and helps to maintain balance and reduce the risk of falling."

"The third strategy to reduce blood pressure is *relaxation*. We have a handout about relaxing breathing exercises or you can pick up a copy of *The Relaxation Response* by Dr. Herbert Benson. This book teaches the importance of breathing exercises to reduce the stress response and lower blood pressure."

At the conclusion of his comprehensive physical examination, David was pensive. "I should have come years ago for regular check-ups. I can't help but wonder if I had been aware of my risk factors earlier and worked to reduce them, I might not have had the heart attack in the first place. That's probably hard to speculate, but starting now, I would like to come in regularly to address my risk factors and other health issues."

Osler's response surprised David. "I agree that preventive health care is important, and I believe that it is more effective to intervene before a catastrophic event rather than afterwards; prevention is cost effective as well as health effective. However, until recently, preventive medicine was not covered by your health insurance. This is why I was pleased that lifestyle counselling was added to the government's medical services plan."

"Does that mean, the government did not pay doctors to get me to quit smoking, lose weight, and learn how to eat right, but will pay for my treatment in an ICU after I have a heart attack? Talk about a false economy! No wonder our health care system is in such a crisis."

"Exactly. That's why this service has now been added[27]. Furthermore, you are more motivated now than you were before your heart attack and therefore more likely to be successful in a lifestyle change. In other words you now realize that if you continue to do what you have always done, you will get more of the same—possibly another heart attack."

David thought about this for a moment. "So how can I get you to help me to improve my lifestyle? I think I can use some effective health coaching, just as my son Adam can use some effective soccer coaching."

Dr. Osler explained that their office provided several uninsured services including preventive health and wellness

---

[27] Personal Health Risk Assessments were added to the British Columbia Medical Services Plan in 2011. As of 2007, the British Columbia government, for the first time, introduced a fee for disease prevention. A cardiac risk analysis became a service which compensated a family physician to discuss cardiovascular disease prevention with a certain number of men and women each year. In January 2011, this was expanded to include lifestyle counselling for smoking, unhealthy eating, physical inactivity, and medical obesity.

counselling. "If you're interested we'll talk about the coaching further after your visit next week. I'll need to check your blood pressure and see how the medication is working, so we'll see you then in any case. In addition, we have referred you to the Cardiac Rehab Program, and its multi-disciplinary team will give you instruction in diet and exercise."

.........................................................................

By the time of the next visit David had eagerly read most of the diet books but found it frustrating there was so much conflicting information. He carried the books with him into the examining room and stacked them on the table. When Dr. Osler came into the room, he greeted David, and after briefly surveying the titles of the stack, he sighed. "I see you have been doing some research; do you have a stack of print outs from the Internet as well? Have you found the perfect diet for yourself?"

David laughed. "That is exactly what I wanted to talk to you about. You recommended the DASH diet for lowering my blood pressure, but I was not sure whether it was an optimal diet for general nutrition or for my heart in particular, so I decided to do some research."

Dr. Osler's reply was thoughtful. "Everyone is different and the same diet is probably not ideal for all people. Individuals need to work within their own parameters regarding tolerance and taste of food, but follow similar nutritional principles. Your confusion is shared by many. Diet books are not necessarily based on solid nutritional principles, and if they all stated the same thing, there would be no market for new books," his physician said dryly.

Then the doctor continued. "To mention just a few examples, the Fit for Life diet advised readers never to eat proteins and carbohydrates together. The Zone Diet recommended the opposite—always eat proteins and carbohydrates and fats together; promising that by eating 30 percent protein, 30 percent fats, and 40 percent carbohydrates you could reach peak performance and ideal health. There have been low-fat diets, then high-protein, high-fat diets, and also low carbohydrate diets. You can Eat Right For Your Type, or try the Palaeolithic Diet or Mediterranean Diet. That only scrapes the surface. Diet books are a huge industry."

"I know the Atkins Diet works. One of the partners in my firm followed it and lost almost fifty pounds," responded David.

Osler sighed. "As you can imagine, a high fat, high animal protein diet is not endorsed by many in the medical profession. The Atkins Diet has been compared to a conventional low-fat diet in a multicenter, randomized, controlled trial. The results, reported in the *New England Journal of Medicine*, showed that the Atkins Diet resulted in greater weight loss by three and six months, but that the difference was not significant at one year. There was also a favourable change in the cholesterol profile in the Atkins group; however, neither group enjoyed the diets long term, and the concluding recommendation was a longer-term study[28]. I believe that in the long run, the best way to lose weight and protect your heart is to eat a varied diet that is low in calories and high in nutrients."

---

[28] Foster, Gary D., et.al, 2003, A Randomized Trial of a Low-Carbohydrate Diet for Obesity, New England Journal of Medicine. 348(21):2082–2090, May 22.

"I simply endorse a sensible meal plan that includes fruits, vegetables, lean protein, healthy fats, and high-fibre complex carbohydrates such as whole grains, nuts and seeds. The focus is on a fresh, preferably organic, mostly in-season diet, including lots of raw plant-based foods. This type of eating is proven to protect heart health and boost weight loss for most people.[29] Personally, I think it's the avoidance of a high glycemic load, not the bacon and fried eggs with cheese that accounted for the benefit of the high fat, high protein diets. But most importantly, any time you restrict calories you will lose weight. And don't forget, David, one of the great pleasures in life is eating. The challenge is eating healthy foods that are also delicious—although it's not as hard as you might have been led to believe."

"Also, be sure to start your day with a good breakfast," Osler reminded his patient. "Too many people skip breakfast as they feel they are too busy getting ready for work, not hungry yet, or wanting to slim down. I recently read a study from Taiwan that gave further evidence that breakfast skippers are twice as likely as breakfast eaters to be obese. More interestingly, however, was that quality of life was studied as well. Not only were the regular breakfast eaters slimmer, they were also happier and more productive!"[30]

---

[29] Chahoud, G., et.al. 2004, Dietary recommendations in the prevention and treatment of coronary heart disease: do we have the ideal diet yet? *The American Journal of Cardiology*, Nov 15;94(10):1260–1267.

[30] Huang, C.J., et al, 2010, Associations of breakfast skipping with obesity and health-related quality of life: evidence from a national survey in Taiwan. Dept. of Anaesthesiology, Buddhist Tzu Chi General Hosp, Taipei, Taiwan, *International Journal of Obesity* (London) 34(4): 720–5 April.

"I'm guilty of breakfast skipping," confessed David. "Now that I don't need to rush to work early in the morning, I can make a point of eating breakfast again, but I'm not sure how I will fit it in when I return to work again."

"I also read a little about the Glycemic Index and Glycemic Load," continued David. "I saw a table listing the GI of various foods. It seems like a complicated way to plan a meal, however."

"It doesn't need to be complicated," Osler replied. "Think of food as fuel for the body. We want to burn oak logs slowly to get even heat rather than throwing newsprint on the fire from time to time. When we take processed carbohydrates such as soft drinks, baked goods containing white flour, or puffed rice and similar products, they immediately raise our blood sugar levels, then insulin rushes in, and the blood sugar levels drop—leaving us craving for more. But worse, the high blood sugar and insulin levels have their own set of problems. The amount of sugar is too much to be used, so some goes into storage as fat. This raises our triglyceride levels, which is a harmful form of cholesterol and therefore increases the risk of heart disease. The high sugar levels increase inflammation in the joints and blood vessels. Furthermore, the high insulin levels lead to insulin resistance, and ultimately to obesity and diabetes."

"So essentially you are saying to avoid white bread?" David asked.

"Correct, white bread does have a high GI, but many healthy-sounding 'multigrain' breads are not much better," Osler advised. "Flour is milled wheat and has a high GI regardless of its colour. Some hearty-looking breads are dark from the added molasses, not whole grains. I have also seen "Organic 12 Grain Nature Bread", which was white bread with a handful of seeds thrown in. Whether it's white or brown, or even whole wheat, your bread needs to pass the squish test."

"Let me guess," David broke in. "If the bread is soft and squishy, the GI is too high, and I should avoid it."

"You're a fast learner, David," Osler grinned. "Good bread is firm and chewy bread. The more whole unprocessed grains, the harder and heavier the bread is."

"So I should avoid white bread, white sugar, saturated fats, and trans fats… anything else?" asked David.

Osler paused for a moment. "If I can get across one point today about diet, it is this: eating is not as much about exclusion as it is about inclusion. Add a variety of unprocessed, unrefined, brightly coloured foods to your diet every day and find flavourful ways to enjoy them. As you make more healthy choices the unhealthy choices will naturally get phased out."

As the appointment ended, David agreed to make concrete plans to improve his diet and do some form of moderate exercise for at least thirty minutes a day, at least five days a week. "I'll follow my elderly German aunt's example," replied David. "She lived by the motto, 'There is no bad weather, only bad clothes' and 'no rest, no rust.'"

Osler smiled. "Sounds like a woman after my own heart."

On his way home, David thought about Osler's practical approach to medicine and his synthesis of information. The appointment had left him feeling more optimistic about the future.

*The practice of medicine is an art, not a trade; not a business, a calling in which your heart will be exercised equally with your head.*

**Sir William Osler**
(1849–1919) Canadian physician and author. The "Father of Modern Medicine" worked at McGill University, Montreal, Quebec, Johns Hopkins University, Baltimore, MD, University of Pennsylvania, Philadelphia, PA, and Oxford University, England.

.........................................................................

David felt that having a health "coach" would be a good thing for him, and allow him to reach his goals more quickly and with greater certainty. But he still found it preposterous that this service was not insured under the government health plan. After all, he was Canadian, and wasn't he therefore entitled to the best comprehensive medical care for free?

.........................................................................

Making an exercise plan was a good motivator for David. Now he needed the tools to put it into action. Back at his apartment, he realized that he had some tasks he shouldn't put off any longer, but he took the time to read a paragraph of 12 Habits.

> " To improve physical activity after a heart attack, use a step counter or pedometer. Most inactive people walk two thousand to four thousand steps a day, whereas

active people walk ten thousand steps or approximately five miles. Start with a fifteen-minute daily walk and increase to a brisk thirty-minute walk at least five times a week. The pedometer can add incentive and track progress. You can even download an app that allows you to chart your distance and do a virtual walk from Vancouver to Halifax, New York to LA, or across Europe.

..................................................................................

The following day, David walked to a fitness store, purchased a pedometer and put it into immediate use. He soon found that his walks increased in length and intensity. He was now doing a brisk thirty-minute walk virtually every day right after he got up. Some days he added a calisthenics routine before his shower. He noticed that after he exercised, his outlook became more positive and that he was beginning to put a little distance between himself and his heart attack. Osler had given him a specific exercise prescription called FITT: Frequency, Intensity, Time, and Type. David's FITT was tailored to his age, physical condition, and medical history:

Frequency: at least four times a week<br>
Intensity: moderate (talking is laboured)<br>
Time: 20–30 minutes<br>
Type: brisk walking, cycling, and swimming

Osler had also told him that when doing endurance exercise, such as running, he should still be able to talk to his running partner. This is something known as the Talk Test, and was found to be a good predictor of one's breathing capacity.[31]

Exercise was one piece of the health equation, but David was also becoming more aware of nutrition now. For instance, what was actually in his favourite breakfast cereal? White flour, sugar, and hydrogenated oil were the first three ingredients listed, followed by a lot of unpronounceable chemical names. It was obviously not the kind of food that was going to nourish him.

David had seen a recipe for muesli in one of his books and headed off to the natural food store to get some ingredients.

**– Methuselah's Marvelous Muesli –**

This recipe can change each time you make it. The idea is to prepare whole grains in a tasty and nutritious manner. Use this as a guideline and improvise according to your own preferences!

**Approximately equal amounts of:**

Organic flakes including: barley, rye, brown rice, triticale, wheat, spelt, kamut—and buckwheat, millet, quinoa, flax seeds, hemp hearts, and chia seeds. (You do not need all of these, but add what you like and vary the recipe.)

**Significantly more:**

Organic oat flakes—go for about half oats and half a mixture of the other grains.

Hard grains (like buckwheat, millet, kamut groats, and in particular, flax) can be ground to make them more digestible.

---

[31] Persinger R., et.al., 2004, Consistency of the Talk Test for exercise prescription. *Medicine and Science in Sports and Exercise*. Sept; 36(9): 1632–6.

Alternately, they can be lightly cooked in your milk of choice or soaked in hot water for a few minutes to soften them. This is then added to the rest of the grains and flakes.

**To this mixture add:**

Various seeds (pumpkin, sunflower, hemp hearts, sesame, chia)
And chopped nuts (almonds, walnuts, hazelnuts)
Dried fruits: raisins, chopped prunes, dates, apricots, cranberries.

**Optional:**

Cinnamon, maple syrup, shredded coconut.

This basic dry mix can be stored at room temperature. (Obviously, if some of the grains have been soaked or ground they will need to be refrigerated.)

**Serve cold:**

Simply take a couple of tablespoons of the mixture and serve with fresh seasonal fruit and either yogurt, kefir, or milk of choice. Additional ground flax, chia, and hemp hearts can be sprinkled on top. It does not need additional sweetening.

**Serve hot:**

Take a few spoonfuls, add more oats, and cook as you would normally make porridge. Top with fresh fruit, ground flax seeds, granola. (If a sweetener is desired, try a little brown sugar, maple syrup, or agave syrup, but the fruit will sweeten it enough).

................................................................................

David was not used to preparing food, and it took him a while to gather and mix the ingredients together, but he did not resent the time. Indeed, he felt proud of his accomplishment and secure in the knowledge that whenever he ate his muesli, he was doing something good for himself.

While at the Good Earth Natural Foods store, David let it slip to the clerk that he recently had a heart attack. "I'm so glad you came," gushed Gail. "I can recommend the supplements you need to restore yourself to good health. And this will be far safer than taking all of the harsh drugs with serious side effects that doctors like to give out."

David accepted her list but decided to run the suggestions by Dr. Osler before taking out a loan to acquire them! He was ready to make a change in his diet but he didn't believe that the word "natural" on a product was necessarily a guarantee that it was good for him. After all, earthquakes and cyanide were natural. So were dandelions, poison ivy, and pond scum; that did not mean they would reduce his risk of heart disease. David enjoyed the enthusiasm of the well-meaning clerk; however, he also appreciated that the supplement industry was big business. Like any expenditure he made, he needed to look into which supplements were most applicable to him and likely to give him a return on his investment. He also wondered how he was going to get through his growing book list when the time came to return to work.

# CHAPTER 4

*"A ship is safe in harbour, but that's not what ships are for."*

**William Shedd**

(1820–1894) American Presbyterian Theologian

David's mother had affectionately called him a "terrier" when he was young because of his determination to succeed in his goals. This quality held him in good stead in his studies and work, but it came with a price. Smoking relieved the tension he felt almost all the time. He had wanted to quit since he started law school but had always found an excuse to continue. He had cut down, but now he realized, he needed to quit completely. Dr. Osler had told him that hard work was required to reduce his risk of having another heart attack. He needed to step out of his comfort zone and not just follow the path of least resistance. It was time to put his dogged determination to good use. David turned once again to *12 Habits.*

*The time is always right to do what is right.*

**Martin Luther King, Jr. (1929–1965)**

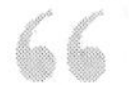

**HABIT THREE: OUT WITH THE BAD**

Often the path to good health can be sabotaged by engaging in practices that are clearly harmful. The most obvious of these is smoking. There is so much evidence that smoking contributes to cancer, heart and lung disease, and many other life worsening and shortening conditions that it defies comprehension that governments allow tobacco products to be sold. The huge amount of taxes raised through the sale of cigarettes does not nearly offset the enormous burden they place on the health care system and society at large. Smoking-relating illnesses kill every

second smoker. Quitting is the single most effective strategy for cutting the risk of many medical conditions.
Smoking adversely affects the cardiac and respiratory systems increasing the risk of heart attacks, irregular heart rate, impaired cardiac function, sudden death, sinusitis, bronchitis, pneumonia, emphysema, asthma, and other lung disease. Smoking dramatically increases peptic ulcer rates, reflux and esophageal cancers. It also increases the risk of osteoporosis and fractures, neurological impairment including stroke, cerebral aneurysms and dementia, along with anxiety and depressive disorders. Smoking worsens chronic kidney disease and immune function and significantly increases the risk of oral, respiratory, reproductive, and digestive cancers, including deadly pancreatic cancers. Female smokers have a higher risk of pelvic inflammatory disease, ectopic pregnancy and infertility. Men who smoke have decreased sperm motility and a higher risk of impotence! Smokers have a suppressed immune system and slower wound healing because of decreased circulation and tissue oxygenation. Smoking is obviously toxic to the fetus resulting in more low-birth-weight babies as well as irritable babies, and it doubles the risk of Sudden Infant Death Syndrome.
In addition, smoking stinks; it causes bad breath, stale smelling hair and clothes, stained teeth and fingernails, and leathery skin. Smokers put themselves at higher risk of injury through fires, motor vehicle accidents, and industrial accidents. It is an expensive, unnecessary habit.
If you smoke, be aware that society offers you more help to quit than ever before. When you are ready to quit—talk to your doctor.

**One minute message**

*Quit smoking* when you are ready and for your own reasons.

Pick a *target date*, buy only one pack at a time, change brands frequently, and smoke only as many cigarettes as you really enjoy. When you are ready to quit, enlist the support of your doctor and friends. Nicotine replacement and other medications can be very helpful.

If there were no benefits to smoking, why would people smoke? The reality is that nicotine from cigarette smoke is one of the most addictive substances known. Nicotine is able to alter the brain chemicals (neurotransmitters) that affect mood. By having a hundred or more puffs a day, each giving a little hit of nicotine, smokers can titrate the levels of these neurotransmitters to feel more alert or more relaxed. This aids in concentration and also allows better coping of everyday stressors. Another factor is that the deep inhalations of cigarette smoke induce a relaxation response by stimulation the parasympathetic nervous system (more on this in Habit Four: Be).

The problem is that along with the nicotine, cigarette smoke contains two thousand or so chemicals, many of them toxic and carcinogenic, which make up the "tar" in the cigarettes. Occupational health inspectors check for many of these chemicals in workplaces, as they pose unacceptable health risks to workers. Yet the same toxins are found in cigarette smoke, where they are legal and unregulated. This is why second hand smoke also contributes a significant risk to one's health. In fact, the recipients of second hand smoke do not have the benefit of the nicotine effects or the advantage of the filter when inhaling side stream smoke. Second hand smoke is the only known toxin that can be legally spewed out on innocent passersby. Many governments now have regulations forbidding smoking in public buildings including hospitals, restaurants, airports, and work places.

To better understand nicotine addiction, a short primer on brain anatomy is helpful. Our human brains are actually a composite of three separate brains. There is the *primitive brain* (also called brain stem) that controls basic unconscious functions such as the drive to breath. Then there is the midbrain, or *emotional brain* (also called the limbic system), and finally, the highly developed *thinking brain* (or cerebral cortex which includes the frontal lobes). As it happens, nicotine stimulates our reptilian brain (brain stem and midbrain)—which is essentially the centre for mood, attention, reward—and addiction. This puts the smoker in conflict between what he or she may *want* to do—stop smoking—and what the reptilian brain is *telling* the person to do: keep smoking. It is important to understand that higher doses of nicotine replacement can be used to tame the cravings and allow the thinking brain to gain the upper hand once again.[32]

Smoking contributes to ill health in multiple body systems, including the gastrointestinal system. Smokers have more indigestion, reflux, and ulcers than do non-smokers. Interestingly, while smoking makes Crohn's Disease

---

[32] Bass, Fred, 2010, Training the inner alligator. *British Columbia Medical Journal*, Vol. 52, No1, Jan/Feb, page 23.

(a form of inflammatory bowel disease—IBD) worse, it has actually been shown to have a beneficial effect on ulcerative colitis (UC is another form of IBD). The reason for this is not clearly understood, however, UC is classically known to get worse with stress. In fact, UC often arises when the body is under stress—even with positive milestones such as job promotions, getting married, buying a house, starting a family or a business. It is therefore quite possible that if smoking is the way one deals with stress, then quitting will make UC flare. *It is very important to be aware of this critical role of stress in our lives, and find ways to mitigate it.* If you stop smoking, and find that you feel worse, it may be the withdrawal symptoms, but it may also be because of a flare in some sort of health condition that has been kept under control with the stress relief obtained by smoking.

Prolonged smoking leads to chronic bronchitis and emphysema, conditions collectively known as COPD (chronic obstructive pulmonary disease). This condition is primarily a result of smoking and is still on the rise as young people are still smoking. Many medications are available to treat this condition, which have been shown to reduce flare ups and hospitalizations: however, once the disease is established, medications will not change the decline in lung function or reduce mortality. Only smoking cessation has been shown to improve lung function and mortality.

To stop smoking, one must make a conscious decision to do so. A person must have the desire to quit—and not feel coerced by someone else. One's readiness and willingness to quit can be gauged by what stage of change they are presently in.

**Stages of Change[33]:**

*Pre-contemplative* (not even thinking about quitting),

*Contemplative* (would like to quit but don't think it will be possible),

*Preparation* (cutting back, changing brands, picking a Target Date to quit),

*Action* (stopping smoking and changing smoke-related behaviours), and

*Maintenance* (finding alternate ways of relaxing and coping with stressors). Unfortunately,

*Relapse* happens from time to time.

Interventions to assist with smoking cessation depend on which of these stages a person is in.

## Tips for quitting:

- ☞ Decide to quit for your own reasons, when you are ready. It is not enough to quit for someone else.
- ☞ Set a Target Date for quitting at least a month away. During this time, taper your consumption of cigarettes gradually to approximately 40–50 percent of current use. Try to pick a date that is meaningful to you such as the birthday of a child or an anniversary. You are more likely to remain true to that date than a random date.
- ☞ Never buy more than one package of cigarettes at a time, and change brands frequently. Most times when one smokes an unfamiliar brand it is less enjoyable, and brings the habit more into consciousness.
- ☞ Do not beat yourself up over the cigarettes you are still smoking, enjoy them! At the same time congratulate yourself for the cigarettes you are not smoking.

---

[33] Prochaska and DiClementi, 1994, *Changing for Good*, in Smoking Reference Section. Also quoted in "Know Smoking" by Dr. Simon Bryant.

☞ Many smokers only enjoy a few cigarettes a day; the rest are consumed as a mindless habit or to restore falling nicotine levels. Try to smoke only the cigarettes you enjoy.

☞ Develop positive mind-speak: In the morning when washing your face, look into the mirror and say; "I am a non-smoker. I may smoke eight cigarettes today because I choose to, but I am a non-smoker and on [Target Date] I will not enjoy smoking anymore and will be free of my addiction." Write down your positive affirmation "I am proud to be a non-smoker" and stick it on your mirror.

☞ As the weeks pass, you will look forward to your quit date with anticipation. The cigarette may have been a good friend, even a best friend, being there for you through thick and thin, but the cigarette is not a true friend. Allow yourself to mourn the loss of the cigarette, but then also rejoice in the end of a bad relationship.

☞ When the quit date arrives, stop smoking. Not even one. While some people can quit cold turkey, quitting is far more successful when combined with nicotine replacement or medications, which help to reduce cravings. Here is where your doctor can help. Good emotional support is also essential during this time.

☞ If you relapse, do not see this as a failure. Understand that you did in fact quit for a length of time, and then determine why you started again. Re-examine your motivation, and prepare to quit again. Remember that most smokers quit numerous times before giving it up for good.

" Most states and provinces have local resources for smoking cessation that are easily found on line. British Columbia offers free smoking cessation counselling and nicotine replacement products to residents—and free information and resources to everyone on the website **Quitnow.ca**. Help is available by phone, on-line, by TXT, and using downloadable tools.

David felt that this was a good time to look up local resources. He had only had a few cigarettes since he was discharged from the hospital but still battled cravings and felt that he did not really have the monkey off his back yet. He already had a target date: Adam's birthday was four weeks away. David knew that Dr. Osler could be enlisted to support him as he began the process.

While moderate consumption of wine may be helpful to one's health (perhaps by causing relaxation in addition to the antioxidant effect), excessive use of alcohol is another significant risk factor for many illnesses. Alcohol is a neurotoxin and has been shown to shrink our brains! Alcoholism, as well as addiction to illicit or prescription drugs, is a disease. The treatment is abstinence following a twelve-step-monitored recovery program. The treatment works if you stick with it. If drugs or alcohol are causing a problem in your life, please attend an Alcoholics Anonymous group and see your doctor.

Other saboteurs are more insidious. Coffee, for example, is a highly addictive substance, which millions of people in our society use to jump-start their day, only to find they fatigue by mid-afternoon. It is a ubiquitous stimulant that activates the sympathetic nervous system leading to anxiety, tremulousness, palpitations, and irritability. It constricts blood vessels, which reduces blood flow to the heart and brain while increasing blood pressure and heart rate. People with hypertension would be well advised to avoid all sources of caffeine.[34] Coffee can cause insomnia even if only one cup is consumed in the morning.

Like most drugs, caffeine has potential benefits as well as harmful side effects. Caffeine can make you feel alert and can help some medications (such as for headaches) work more quickly and effectively. Coffee has no calories and no fat and the stimulant effect may help with weight loss. Proponents point out that coffee may be beneficial for Alzheimer's disease, diabetes, and liver disease, as well as skin cancer. The blood pressure elevation might be helpful to seniors who have sluggish circulation.

However, coffee irritates the stomach lining and contributes to acid reflux. In addition, coffee can aggravate the prostate gland and cause breast pain. The stimulating effect fools you into thinking that you have had enough sleep. Research suggests it also may cause calcium loss through urine, which can contribute to the formation of kidney stones. A recent study concluded that drinking just two cups of coffee per day may increase the risk of kidney stone formation in people with a history of the condition.[35] Calcium loss also can weaken bones and affect nerve impulse transmission, blood pressure regulation, and muscle contraction. Excess caffeine

---

[34] Farag, N.H., et.al., 2005, Caffeine tolerance is incomplete: persistent blood pressure responses in the ambulatory setting. *American Journal of Hypertension* May; 18(5 Pt 1):714–719.

[35] Massey, L.K., Sutton, R. A., 2004, Acute caffeine effects on urine composition and calcium kidney stone risk in calcium stone formers. *The Journal of Urology*, Aug; 172(2):555–8.

consumption is inadvisable for people with a history of anxiety, nervousness, tremor, and insomnia.

A delay in raising one's caffeine levels to therapeutic thresholds in the morning results in irritability and a pounding headache. Many chronic health problems can be reduced by eliminating the daily use of coffee.

It is also important to reduce exposure to toxins from our food and personal care products. The skin is our largest organ and serves as a semi-permeable membrane. That is, our body can absorb a lot of substances through the skin. Many medications including hormones, nicotine, nitroglycerin, and narcotic analgesics are delivered through patch therapy. The skin can also absorb substances directly from the air or water. Knowing this, it is important to check shampoos, antiperspirants, and lotions for potentially harmful ingredients.

While conventional farmers have done extremely well to feed a growing population efficiently, the use of pesticides and herbicides is a significant health concern. The toxicity of many of these chemicals is additive and the combinations have not been adequately evaluated. There is no doubt that prolonged exposure increases the risk of cancer and impairs fertility. Moreover, just as overuse of antibiotics leads to resistance and the development of "superbugs", the heavy use of pesticides results in greater problems with insect infestations. It is important to choose organically grown soft-skinned fruits, such as strawberries, peaches, apricots, and grapes, as these are among the most contaminated.

As developing organisms are more susceptible to the toxic effects of these chemicals, it is especially prudent to seek organically grown foods for infants and children.

Children are probably also more vulnerable to toxic effects of radiation. While it is impossible in a civilized society to avoid exposure to electromagnetic, microwave, and wireless communication devices, the radiation from these sources could pose significant health risks, especially to those most vulnerable. This type of pollution is all the more insidious as it is virtually invisible. Consider these factors when choosing where to live (avoid proximity to high voltage power lines), and how to cook your food (stop nuking food in microwave ovens—especially in plastic containers). Be wary of screening radiographs (especially CT scans, now thought to account for two percent of cancers). If you have no symptoms work with your physician to evaluate the risks and benefits of diagnostic tests.

We are also exposed to background radiation that comes from the earth (mainly radon gas). One trans-Atlantic flight over the North Pole results in the equivalent radiation to a chest x-ray. Heavy metal and nuclear contamination is found in land and sea. Clearly, we cannot avoid all sources of radiation and toxicity, yet they need to be considered when looking at the multiple causes of illness, in particular cancer and degenerative conditions.

..................................................................................

David glumly put the book down. "Wow, I need to get unplugged and move into the wilderness!" He didn't see his alcohol consumption as a problem, although he enjoyed a good bottle of red wine when out for dinner, and the occasional beer or scotch at home in the evening. However, his day would just not be the same without that "hot cuppa java" first thing in the morning, and a few more throughout the day. Yes, he had noticed that on the rare occasions he went without coffee he would develop a pounding headache, but that could be easily remedied with another quick cup and a couple of aspirin. Yes, he was a restless sleeper but that was probably due to other stresses in his life. He sometimes got heartburn with a sour taste in his mouth, but surely that couldn't be blamed entirely on his coffee consumption.

It struck him suddenly that it was a habit, and not necessarily a good one. In fact, he reasoned, since he was having withdrawal symptoms, he must be addicted to the stuff! If he really was going to make an effort to extend his warranty, as Osler put it, then he was going to have to break some of his bad habits and adopt some new ones. Maybe he would give green tea a try. He had read somewhere that it was a healthier choice, and it still had caffeine in it to give him a boost.

Back to his action plan for quitting smoking. He vaguely remembered hearing that heart patients should not use nicotine replacement therapy. He flipped back to the smoking section of Habit 3 and read:

> It is more dangerous for patients with heart disease to continue to smoke than to use nicotine replacement. Given the seriousness of their medical condition, cardiac patients who cannot quit smoking should be among those first considered for nicotine replacement or medications that may reduce cravings.
>
> It is extremely dangerous for patients with heart disease to continue to smoke. Smoking causes the activation

of clotting pathways and the promotion of clot formation, which can cause heart attacks. A cardiac patient who smokes also exposes himself to significant heart toxins such as carbon monoxide and gases that reduce oxygen delivery to the heart. The role of tobacco in causing heart disease is primarily by toxins making up the "tar" rather than nicotine. The stimulant effect of nicotine may, however, aggravate cardiovascular disease and therefore use of any of these treatments must be based upon an assessment of the potential risks and benefits of treatment.

David decided the sensible thing to do was to discuss this issue with Osler. He also realized he hadn't yet phoned the number on the business card to return *12 Habits*, but he hoped the person who'd left it could wait a few more days. Then, he thought with a smile, he'd be able to give the owner a full book review.

# CHAPTER 5

*"We cannot see our reflection in running water—it is only in still water that we can see."*

**Zen expression**

It had probably been there for years but David had never noticed it before. A short bike ride from his apartment David had discovered the Peninsula Athletic Club. He had been walking and cycling almost daily and felt the difference now that he had started to get some physical exercise. He now wanted to commit to pushing himself a little harder and decided to check out this local gym.

David parked his bike near the front door and climbed the stairs to the entrance. As he opened the front door he was greeted by the subtle but familiar smell of chlorine. When he was growing up he had swum a lot at the YMCA and through their Junior Leaders program had also taught younger kids how to swim. In high school and college David had played on water polo teams, and those happy memories came back as he approached the front counter.

A fit young woman with auburn hair and green eyes smiled at him pleasantly from behind the counter. She was wearing a crisp white golf shirt with the name of the club embroidered on the left side. "Welcome to the Peninsula Club. How may I help you, sir?" asked Victoria.

David asked her about the services the club offered, as well as its hours of operation and fees. After answering his queries, Victoria arranged for another staff member to show David around.

Jamie, who looked to be about David's age and build, although about 30 pounds slimmer, was wearing a tracksuit smartly emblazoned with the "PAC" logo. He showed David the fitness centre complete with rows of exercise bicycles, treadmills, elliptical cross trainers, stair climbers, rowing ergometers, weight machines, free weights, and cardiac monitors. Here and there personal trainers instructed people on equipment use and guided them through individualized fitness programs. David and Jamie also toured the hardwood gymnasium, Olympic-sized swimming pool, squash courts, running track on the roof, and the executive changing rooms and spa facilities.

Dr. Schreiber at the hospital had told him he would be attending a cardiac rehab program as an important part of his recovery and to reduce his risk of a subsequent heart attack. Although David felt that by joining the Peninsula Club immediately, he would have a head start on that program, he did feel it prudent to clear it with Osler first.

David met with his physician during the following week. They chatted about cardiac rehab, how his diet was going, his exercise program, and smoking cessation. Dr. Osler challenged David to be more specific when he was reporting his progress back to him. "I serve on the Quality and Safety committee at St. Luke's," said the physician. "Our mantra in Quality Improvement is 'If you don't measure it, you can't improve it.' So I would like you to start measuring a few things and chart them in a personal health log. You will need a blood pressure monitor and a heart rate monitor in addition to your pedometer. These are sound investments in your health."

"Calculate your aerobic target heart rate," instructed the doctor. "Take 220, subtract your age to get your maximum heart rate. Then calculate 60–80 percent of the max as your target range. Write this range down, memorize it, and recalculate it every year. I would like you to get a journal—our diabetic patients do this for their blood sugar readings—and mark down the date, how many minutes you exercised and at what heart rate. You can also record the distances you walk when you wear your pedometer. You could log what type of exercise you did that day, especially when you start weight training. How many pounds and how many reps? I also want you to measure and write down your BP twice a day. Journal the number of cigarettes you smoke each day. Record your weight every week; it's not necessary to weigh yourself every day as minor fluctuations do not matter."

He continued, "You may also want to use your personal health log to plan some active holidays. Try to get away once a month for a mental health and fitness break, which may be a six-hour hike on the North Shore, a kayak trip around Salt Spring Island, or a cycling tour through Napa Valley or the Pyrenees!"

David thought this advice was far more detailed than he wanted, but Dr. Osler reminded him that coaches work with athletes to improve their performance in sports; he was coaching David to improve and prolong his life. "The journal will hold you accountable to yourself and will be an easy way for me to assess your progress every few weeks."

David then asked him what he thought about vitamins and other supplements. Dr. Osler answered that he took a few supplements himself but felt strongly that most of our nutrients are available through a healthy diet. He added that he was more likely to take additional vitamins when he was away from his own kitchen and routine. Osler pointed out that in his experience, people who took vitamins regularly were also the most health conscious about eating right and exercising.

"On the other hand, some of the homeless folks and alcoholics who show up in our ER are quite malnourished and are the ones that benefit most from vitamin supplements. In fact, they are given thiamine and folic acid—which are B vitamins—daily as well as IV multivitamins to reduce the occurrence of a neurological syndrome and anaemia. Some of our ER nurses disparagingly refer to the golden IV infusion as the "Bag of Shame," but I think IV vitamins are a great idea for many people who are recovering from surgery or fighting an infectious illness."

Seeing that David was listening intently, Osler continued. "Antioxidant vitamins have not been as effective in clinical trials as one would think based on their antioxidant effect in the lab.[36] I suspect a reason is that the effect is blunted by the digestive system. I'm sure there is abundant benefit in regularly ingesting antioxidant foods and supplements, but in times of illness, the effect is much more potent when they are given intravenously."

"How many vitamins does the average person need?" asked David.

"Many vitamins are essential enzymes and co-factors for biochemical reactions in the body," replied Osler, pleased that his new patient showed such a willingness to learn. "However, they are required in small amounts that can generally be derived from a healthy diet." He paused for a moment. "Remember that the word is 'supplement' not 'replacement.' These substances work best when taken in addition to a healthy diet, not instead of it. It is a mistake to consume a diet of fast, processed foods and feel that any missing nutrients can be replaced in pill form. However, it makes sense to supplement the substances we can't get enough of on a daily basis."

---

[36] Packer, Lester, et. al, 1999, *The Antioxidant Miracle*, New York, John Wiley & Sons, Inc., details studies from his laboratory demonstrating the potent antioxidant effect of several vitamins and phytochemicals. Many clinical trials have been done using vitamin supplements. Some of these compared a combination of vitamins to a placebo and in other trials individual vitamins (such as Vitamin E) were added as an arm in a medication trial to determine their effect against heart disease. Some of these trials have proven that the addition of multivitamins reduces the rate of certain cancers, but several of the larger trials have been disappointing. It would be great to have solid evidence proving that by simply popping a vitamin pill we can dramatically lower the risk of heart disease, cancer, dementia, and other serious health conditions. Unfortunately, this reductionist thinking is not scientifically based, nor is it logical. Despite good evidence that several vitamins have an antioxidant effect in the laboratory, taking them in isolation may not improve overall health. However, these supplements are safe and when combined with a healthy lifestyle probably have significant benefits despite randomized clinical trials not reaching statistical significance.

"Right now, the most evidence-based supplement is Vitamin D, which our bodies make by exposure to sunlight," said Osler. "So while sunburns increase the risk of skin cancer, sunlight increases Vitamin D levels and reduces the risk of several cancers, multiple sclerosis, fractures, falls, hypertension, diabetes, psoriasis, and some infections. In addition, it strengthens our muscles and immune system, may reduce chronic pain and cognitive decline, and has been shown to reduce overall mortality from all causes, and cancer mortality in particular.[37] Here in British Columbia we do not get a lot of sunshine in the winter months, so I make sure to take more Vitamin D then."

"I also think that essential fats from fish oils are very important for health and may not be obtained from our diet on a daily basis. There are indications of benefit from the cradle to the grave. These supplements are now recommended for pregnant woman and newborns for brain and eye development and may be helpful for improved attention and focus in school aged kids. They are certainly of benefit to the heart and joints and may help with cognitive functioning in seniors. They help reduce the risk of age-related macular degeneration (a leading cause of blindness in seniors) and are effective for post-partum and clinical depression."

Many of Dr. Osler's patients only seemed to want a prescription filled. David, however, appeared to be an eager student of the science of medicine. "In addition to Vitamin D and fish oils, I think that adding some plant sterols is a good idea for men like you, David, with a cardiac history. They have been shown to lower

---

[37] Bosomworth, N.J., 2011, Mitigating epidemic vitamin D deficiency, *Canadian Family Physician*, Vol. 57, January, p 16–20

cholesterol, are not expensive, and may benefit your prostate gland as well. So those are three supplements that I can recommend."

"Because you take a statin drug, which we know depletes your body's levels of Coenzyme Q10, I would support you taking a CoQ10 supplement as well. In addition, a broad spectrum multivitamin that has little or no iron is a good insurance policy for you to take daily, along with a small amount of vitamin C twice a day. Along with aspirin and your prescription meds, I think that's a reasonable as well as an affordable list," said Osler.

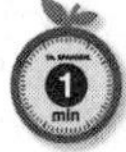


**One minute message**

A few *nutritional supplements* are important in addition to a healthy diet, as some essential nutrients are not sufficiently available on a daily basis.

*Vitamin D* and *Omega -3 Fatty Acids* are safe, effective, and inexpensive. They are recommended for pregnant and lactating women, infants and children undergoing rapid growth and development, adolescents, adults with joint problems, heart disease, macular degeneration, and neurological conditions. Regular usage has been shown to reduce cancer and degenerative conditions and to stabilize moods. In short, everyone would benefit from these supplements for the prevention or treatment of multiple conditions.

David was feeling a lot more comfortable about the whole issue of supplements, but had other concerns that he wanted to run past his doctor. "I'm a bit worried about electromagnetic radiation," he began. "It's all around us from power lines to cell phones, electronic devices, and wireless Internet connections. I had never given it much thought before, but I read it could be a very significant problem. What are your thoughts, Doc?"

"I think that people who suffer from electro-hypersensitivity may be the canaries in the coal mine," Osler answered. "I sometimes have patients tell me they get headaches, fatigue, nausea, and palpitations around various wireless devices, and while it is difficult to prove that these devices are harmful, it is not hard to imagine that they may have an effect on susceptible individuals. We know that most people have no adverse effects from silver mercury dental fillings, for example, yet some patients feel better when they have them removed. In the same way, certain people may be more sensitive to the radiation that we are all exposed to. Personally, I shun microwave ovens, and try to use devices that are hard wired as well as checking for high voltage lines and transformers near areas where I live and work."

Peter Osler also wanted to know how David coped with his demanding job and having a young family to support. David had never talked to a professional about "stress" before. Sure, he worked a lot of late nights, and yes, he and Jessica were separated at the moment, but he was still a good dad. Stress was just a normal part of life. After all, things could be worse. If anyone could cope, he could. Whenever he had any injuries or expressed any fears as a child, his father would tell him to shake it off and suck it up—so that's what he had always done.

"I do feel vulnerable and afraid, though," David admitted slowly. "I worry, especially now that I've had the heart attack, that if I die, my children will lose a role model and not reach their potential. I worry that Jessica and I may not get back together. But if I don't spend sixteen hours a day at my work, how can I get ahead? It's a very competitive field."

Dr. Osler had noticed that it is always harder to motivate change when status quo is acceptable. It is only when present circumstances are bleak that change can occur. The doctor enjoyed the challenge of doing Health and Wellness coaching as it allowed him to spend more time to effect permanent change in people's lives. Unfortunately, this was simply not possible within the constraints of regular office appointments.

Osler suggested that he see David on a regular basis, initially once a month, and give him the opportunity to work with other professionals as required. He would also help David set goals and priorities and assist him in achieving them.

Dr. Osler informed David that copies of his clinical records from St. Luke's had arrived, and that his last stress test had showed no worrisome changes. Dr. Schreiber had thereby cleared him for cardiac rehabilitation treatment. During this program, his heart rate would be monitored while he exercised.

"One more question, Dr. Osler," asked David. "I'd like to join the Peninsula Club and get a head start on the cardiac rehab. What are your thoughts?"

"I think you will benefit from the supervised exercise program at the cardiac rehab centre," replied Osler, "but as you did not have significant heart damage, I feel you can certainly start doing some stretching and light exercises on your own or with a trainer at the club. Just remember the motto to 'start low and go slow,' and stop if you develop any chest discomfort."

As a nutritional exercise, Dr. Osler asked David to come up with his own "Top Ten" list of foods. Dr. Osler told him that in other sessions, in addition to information on diet and exercise, they would spend time on topics such as effective relaxation techniques, the need to be curious and learn new things, the importance of spending time in peaceful places, seeking out inspirational people, and forgiving those individuals who may have hurt him in the past.[38]

David's head was spinning by the end of their session, as he felt that for the first time that he was on a path to wellness. Strange as it seemed, he almost felt grateful for his illness, in that it had given him the opportunity to put his life into perspective. He was confident that by the end of this process, he would, in many ways be healthier than he had been before his heart attack.

When David left, Dr. Osler reflected as to how he could better motivate other patients to change their behaviour. He had studied philosophy during his undergraduate days and was inspired by the ancient Greek philosophers. Socrates believed that teaching did not need to involve a lot of telling. As long as one asked the right questions, a student could use his or her intelligence to discover the truth. Thus the questions became a means of stimulating critical thinking. Osler wanted to become a more effective teacher because it was obvious that simply telling patients to stop smoking or start exercising did not work.

---

[38] Weil, Andrew, 1997, *8 Weeks to Optimum Health*, Alfred A. Knopf, New York, outlines a practical, step-wise approach to improving health by making positive lifestyle changes.

*Quieting the mind quiets the body, and the less turbulent the body is, the more the self-repair healing mechanisms get amplified. In fact, scientists have shown that the better your DNA, your genetic machinery is at healing itself, the longer you live. That's how meditation lowers biological age.*

**Deepak Chopra**

(1946– ) physician and author of many books on spirituality, mind-body medicine, and Ayurveda—the traditional medicine of India.

---

**HABIT FOUR: BE**

Early man spent a lot of time just "being." Of course, he had to hunt and gather, find shelter and make clothes and fire or he would not survive, but there were a lot of times when groups of men, women, and children would sit around, play, or watch the clouds. In addition, with no electricity, they also slept a lot more than is the custom today.

Our civilization then moved into the Industrial Age of "doing." The focus was on production and division of labour. This pattern continues to the present, combining with the phenomenon of "having." Doing and having now occupy most of our time.

Remember that we are human "beings," not human "doings" or "wanting." Our emotional, physical and even financial success depends on us to "Be" first, then to "Do" and then to "Have." Too often people feel they need to *have* wealth and possessions, in order to *do* things they want to so that they can *be* who they want to be.

Consider another approach: everything starts with the mind. First conceive of who and what you wish to *be*, and then *do* the things that need to be done, until you ultimately have what it is you need and want. You may not end up getting everything that you think you want—but you will likely achieve the things that you need and that resonate with who you are.

Meditation—which sounds a lot like medication as the words have the same origin—is a practice that helps to quiet and focus the mind and allows us to spend more time "being." Anyone can learn it. Dr. Jon Kabat-Zinn points out that meditation is like tuning an instrument.[39] Our minds need to be tuned to function optimally. Meditation is about being mindful and present as we go about our lives. This "awareness" allows us to "*be*" even while we "*do*."

**Mindfulness means remaining in the present moment**—on purpose. Focus on becoming aware of yourself—your breathing, your emotions, and your thoughts—all with non-judgmental acceptance. Observe yourself breathing, and observe your thoughts and emotions without trying to change them. This kind of attention nurtures greater awareness, clarity, and acceptance of the present. *Mindfulness* can be a helpful

---

[39] Kabat-Zinn, J., PhD, a practitioner and teacher of yoga since the 1960s is the author of *Full Catastrophe Living: Using the Wisdom of Your Body and Mind to Face Stress, Pain, and Illness*, Delta, 1990, and *Wherever You Go, There You Are: Mindfulness Meditation in Everyday Life*, Hyperion, 1994.

strategy for managing insomnia, pain, and depression, and can be used to improve performance on tasks that require focus. According to Professor Ellen Langer, a *mindful* approach has three characteristics: 1. the continuous creation of new categories, 2. openness to new information, and 3. an implicit awareness of more than one perspective.[40]

Being "mindless," on the other hand, is being set in our ways and not open to new alternatives. It can be compared to being on auto-pilot in a car: doing things as we have always done them, and sometimes not even aware of what we are doing.

This is *life-altering stuff*, David thought. Yet it made sense and on some level he already knew about the concept—he just needed to live it. As he thought about his work, the next few paragraphs hit home.

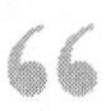

To enjoy abundant health, it is important to take time to relax. This means taking short breaks throughout the day to collect one's thoughts, as well as planning regular vacations. Vacations recharge our batteries, and allow us to develop ideas and thoughts that do not enter into our minds when we are busy.

An effective way to relax is to focus on the present. Worries about the past and anxieties about future challenges prevent us from focusing on the present. These distracting thoughts need to be gently dismissed

---

[40] Langer, E., 1989, *Mindfulness*, and 1997, *The Power of Mindful Learning*, published by Addison-Wealey, Reading, Massachusetts.

from consciousness. Breathing is always in the present, so it is the best possible starting point. This includes observing oneself breathe, much as one watches a sleeping child or waves in the ocean rise and fall. It also includes altering the depth and rate of our breath in order to effect physiological change.

Normally, our breathing is shallow and comes mainly from chest expansion. When we feel anxious or stressed, breathing becomes faster and shallower. Relaxing breathing, on the other hand is slower and deeper. It comes from lowering the diaphragm and breathing into the belly. The act of taking a deep breath stimulates the parasympathetic nervous system, which begins to induce a calming effect in the body. Practice "belly breathing" by putting your hand on your abdomen at the level of the belly button. Take a slow deep breath, like blowing up a balloon in your tummy and feel your hand rise. (You may need to push your belly out into your hand to feel it the first time.) Then blow out slowly and feel your hand fall again (or push your hand into your abdomen to empty your lungs). When practising breathing exercises, breathe in and out of your belly—feeling your abdomen rise and fall while your hand moves out and in. This is how singers and musicians who play brass or wood wind instruments breathe to get through long phrases. They do not throw their shoulders back and gasp into their chest, but take a long breath into the belly by lowering their diaphragm.

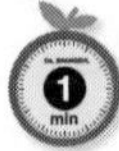

**One minute message**

Our bodies are capable of both a Stress Response and a Relaxation Response. Either one could be life saving in the appropriate setting. The Stress Response ("fight or flight") is innate; the Relaxation Response ("rest and digest") is learned.

To induce relaxation, *breathe in* through your nose to the count of four. *Hold* for the count of seven, and then *breathe out* your mouth in a sigh to the count of eight. Four breaths like this are usually enough.

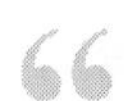

The *autonomic nervous system*, so named as it is "independent" of our conscious mind, works in the background without our thinking about it. It is divided into the *sympathetic and parasympathetic* branches. The sympathetic nervous system is involved in the "fight or flight" response; the changes that occur under times of stress, when early man needed to fight to stay alive, or run away to escape from danger. Today's stressors, for the most part, are less physically frightening than sabre-toothed tigers, yet our body's responses are the same. Our senses are heightened as our bodies prepare for battle: we may feel worried or anxious or even filled with a sense of foreboding or doom. Stress hormones such as adrenaline and cortisol rise. Our heart rate and blood pressure rise, blood clots more easily, and blood flow is directed to the muscles and away from the digestive organs. At the same time, breathing becomes rapid and shallow. This "stress response" is innate; that is we are born with this system hard wired into our bodies. It may have allowed our ancestors to survive in tough times. Yet, the stress response, while still beneficial for soldiers in battle and for some competitors, is largely no longer helpful to us. A certain amount of stress does improve performance just as a certain amount of anxiety is needed to be wary of strangers and risky situations. However, too much of the stress response can manifest itself as an anxiety disorder, cause insomnia or hypertension, damage our blood vessels, and increase our risk of stroke and heart disease.

The parasympathetic branch of the autonomic nervous system, on the other hand, fulfils the "rest and digest" functions. It slows the heart rate and respiration, improves intestinal and glandular activity and relaxes muscular sphincters. These digestive and regulatory functions can offset the changes brought on by the sympathetic nervous system. Thus, the simple act of taking a deep breath can cause profound physiological changes in the body that lead to a feeling of relaxation. This "relaxation response" is available for everyone to benefit from. However, unlike the stress response, this simple technique must be learned.[41]

With deep, abdominal breathing, the downward and upward movements of the diaphragm, combined with the outward and inward movements of the belly and lower ribcage help to massage the stomach, liver, intestines, and heart. This, along with the stimulation of parasym-

---

[41] Benson, H., 1975, *The Relaxation Response,* New York: William Morrow and Co. This was one of the first medically validated books to discuss the role of breathing in relaxation and in lowering blood pressure in particular.

pathetic nerves—mainly the vagus and phrenic nerves—improves digestion and relaxation. Deep breathing also promotes blood flow and regular contractions of the bowel, and pumps the lymph more efficiently through our lymphatic system. Deeper respiration also improves tissue oxygenation and helps blow off carbon dioxide. Excess $CO^2$ levels result in "brain fog"—making us feel tired and sluggish. Improved respiration is a key advantage to aerobic exercise; however, it can also be achieved safely and effectively by practising deep abdominal breathing. This is particularly helpful for people who suffer from respiratory illnesses such as asthma and chronic lung disease (bronchitis and emphysema). Patients with irregular heart rates can be taught to stimulate their parasympathetic nervous system by doing a Valsalva Maneuver. This involves taking a deep breath, holding it, and then bearing down in a similar way to having a bowel movement. The increased intra-abdominal pressure stimulates the parasympathetic nervous system and slows down the heart or corrects the rhythm.

Yogic deep-breathing techniques (pranayama) combined with yogic postures (asanas) along with meditation have been found to be effective in treating a wide range of clinical conditions including stress, anxiety, and depression. These techniques enhance wellbeing, mood, attention, mental focus, and stress tolerance, and should be considered as a low-risk, low-cost, beneficial adjunct, or substitute for the treatment of many health conditions.[42] Slow, deep rhythmic breathing which can stimulate the parasympathetic nervous system and turn on the relaxation response should be practised for even a few minutes each day. There are numerous breathing exercises that are helpful, but a great place to start is with an age-old breathing pattern practiced in yoga. To do this exercise, place the tongue in "yogic position," with the tip touching the alveolar ridge—the gum tissue directly behind where the front teeth are rooted. The tongue remains in this forward position throughout the entire exercise, while breathing in and out. Start the exercise by breathing in through your nose for the count of *four*, then hold for the count of *seven*, then exhale in a slow sigh past the tongue for the count of *eight*. Usually, four slow cycles of this pattern are sufficient to induce a comfortable state of relaxation. Practising this technique first thing in the morning and before falling asleep, will help to balance the autonomic nervous system and produce significant relaxation and additional health benefits. Also, by practising regularly, you will more reliably be able to induce a relaxation response when you are in a stressful situation.

Meditation has been shown to help reduce blood pressure and heart rate as well as other markers of physiological and psychological stress. It is also helpful in focusing the mind and instilling a sense of well-being and inner peace. Meditation can also be a useful treatment of many diseases, including heart disease, and also in particular autoimmune conditions in which the body makes antibodies to its own proteins.

---

[42] Brown, Richard, and Gerbarg, Patricia, 2005, published a two-part review article on the benefits of yoga for mental health: Sudarshan Kriya Yogic Breathing in the Treatment of Stress, Anxiety, and Depression: Part II—Clinical Applications and Guide. *The Journal of Alternative and Complementary Medicine*. August, 11(4): 711–717.

Psoriasis is a poorly understood condition in which there is abnormal, but non-cancerous proliferation and thickening of the skin. A variety of medications are used to control it, and dietary interventions and moisturizing of the skin are also important. The condition is typically improved with exposure to sunlight (perhaps through the role of Vitamin D "the sunshine vitamin" which can also be applied topically in cream form). Studies comparing ultra-violet light therapy alone with light therapy and meditation have found a four-fold improvement in the group that also meditated.

Anyone with a chronic illness would be well advised to practise meditation; often there is some improvement in the condition, and sometimes a significant reduction in the medications needed to control the symptoms. When combined with a nutritious diet and healthy lifestyle, the results can be dramatic. Being present in meditation also results in a certain acceptance of the chronic condition, which makes it more tolerable.

Regular practice of meditation has been shown to activate specific brain chemicals which sharpen the mind, improve energy, as well as relaxation and sleep. It leads to better resilience to stress, and a slowing in the biological markers of aging. For example, HGH (human growth hormone) and DHEA (dehydroepiandrosterone) and melatonin levels rise with meditation, and cortisol (a stress hormone) levels decline.

Meditation helps to improve concentration, and by focusing on the present can bring the body into consciousness. In a society fraught with attention deficit disorder, and preoccupation with the past and the future, meditation can reduce distractibility and reclaim the present. In this way, body, mind, and spirit can be brought into harmony.

**To experience the benefits of meditation:**

1. Find a relaxing and quiet location. Eliminate distractions such as telephones or pagers and give yourself permission to spend twenty to thirty uninterrupted minutes by yourself.

2. Assume a comfortable sitting position in a chair or on the floor. One can also meditate when walking or lying down. If you fall asleep when meditating, it only means you are not getting enough sleep. Try again when you are more alert. Focus the mind by remaining in the present. Visualize a peaceful scene, a garden, a quiet pond, or a forest trail while letting your breath go in and out. Repeating a phrase, word or sound—called a mantra—helps to focus attention and slow thinking for mental clarity. It can interrupt the stress response and transform consciousness. The vibrations that result from the spoken word as well as their meaning and intention can be therapeutic.

3. Consider gazing at a flame, plant, or meaningful object. This may help to keep distracting thoughts from entering your consciousness. It is normal for the mind to wander—it's how the mind works—it does not mean that you are not meditating. Allow thoughts that enter to leave again and recognize

that as you practise, your mind will gradually become quieter. Also understand that you are not your mind. Your mind is a tool, much like your eye or your hand. Therefore, we need to learn to control it. We are the thinkers of our thoughts, but we are not our thoughts. As an exercise sit quietly and see what thoughts cross your mind without you putting them there. See how long your mind allows silence before filling it with another thought. Sit like a cat watching a mouse hole and "catch" the next thought that comes out.

4. Adopt a passive attitude. Be aware of your breath moving in and out of your body without influencing it. Surf the feeling of the breath as it rolls rhythmically in and out —like waves on a shore. Follow these natural breathing movements and allow yourself to simply "be." Being still and setting the mind on "receive" and not always "send" can be the source of great inspiration and unexpected insights.

5. Understand that while relaxation will occur quickly, other health benefits may not be obvious immediately. Be patient and persistent; commit to long-term practice.

6. Smile when you meditate; adopt an *attitude of gratitude*. Being grateful improves focus and happiness. Each day, reflect on three things that you are grateful for. This can be as simple as the air you breathe, a flower you walk by, the warmth of the sun, family, or friends, or any of your countless gifts and talents.

David put down the book. He had always believed that meditation was something complicated and spiritual practised by monks in the Far East who never spoke to anybody. He had also suspected that because it wasn't "productive," it was essentially a waste of time. Who knew there were health benefits?

As he was comfortably curled up on the couch, he felt it would not hurt to try the "four, seven, eight thing," So he touched the tip of his tongue to the gums behind his front teeth and closed his eyes. He took a deep breath in through his nose as he counted slowly to four. He held his breath for the count of seven, and then let out a long sigh for the count of eight, pursing his lips slightly, with his tongue still touching the same spot on his gums. He did this four times. He was a little lightheaded but felt surprisingly content. He did not open his eyes for a few moments, but sat quietly enjoying the feeling.

David realized that he had been wallowing in self-pity since his accident and blamed Jessica for turning her back on him when he needed her the most. He put all that aside and became aware of his breathing and his emotions without trying to change them. David smiled—and felt grateful for the things that were good in his life. He had survived his heart attack and had been given a second chance to lead a healthy life. He had an interesting and rewarding job; he had two terrific kids; and if he wanted to mend the relationship with their mother, that would be up to him.

When he opened his eyes, David remembered that Joanna Lee from the firm was dropping by that afternoon to discuss some of their cases. With a newborn sense of relaxation, he looked forward to their meeting. He would just have time to tidy up the apartment and put on the kettle before she arrived.

# CHAPTER 6

*We ourselves feel that what we are doing is just a drop in the ocean. But the ocean would be less because of that missing drop.*

**Mother Teresa of Calcutta**

(1910–1997) Albanian nun and founder of the Missionaries of Charity in India, an international religious order.

As David walked into the Peninsula Club he saw a familiar face at the juice bar fuelling up on something green that came from a blender. "Sister Mary Ann! The Angel of Mercy from St. Luke's!" he teased.

It took her only a moment to recognize her previous patient. "Hello David!" the nurse replied. "I hardly recognized you outside the hospital. Do you come here often?"

"Actually, I just joined," he explained. "I have had my stress test, but the cardiac rehab program does not start until next week. I was going a bit stir crazy at home, so I decided to get some fresh air and exercise. I thought I would ease into it slowly with a light swim, and then I was thinking of taking in a qi-gong or yoga class. I've never done that before, but I was recently reading about the benefits of relaxation therapy and breathing exercises."

"There's a yoga class starting in fifteen minutes," Mary Ann informed him. "Why don't you skip the swim and join me? Besides, I'd hate to see you drown when you are just beginning to make such progress down the road to recovery."

They chatted briefly about different kinds of yoga including Power Yoga or Ashtanga yoga, and Bikram Yoga, (which takes place in a heated studio) before entering the yoga studio for a beginner class in Hatha Yoga. "This is physical yoga." said Mary Ann. "Several poses and movements are used to improve flexibility and strength, at the same time as you become aware of breathing and achieving relaxation."

A wiry but muscular man with a clean shaven head and engaging smile walked into the studio. He was of South Asian descent and looked as if he were in his early forties, although he may have been twenty years older than he looked. "My name is Johnny Sharasna, and it is my pleasure to guide you through your class today." (David had already seen Johnny around the Club; he had the peculiar habit of bending down and touching his forehead to his knee.)

Johnny asked the students to focus on their breathing and listen carefully to his dialogue as he led them through a series of postures. "Concentrate, meditate—and begin," were the simple words he used. Although there were some advanced students in class who had the propensity to twist themselves into pretzels, David, a beginner, was told that maximum benefit from each posture would occur just by attempting the set-up as deliberately as possible. In many cases, dynamic stretches were practised when one's own strength was required to go deeper into the stretch.

David found the class tough. He was self-conscious about the fact that he had just suffered a heart attack in his early forties. He felt stiff and awkward trying even the most basic moves. At the end of the class, he did feel some relaxation when he could simply lie on his back and breath, using a posture aptly named the "Corpse Pose."

Mary Ann told him after the session that even a single yoga class can lower the amount of cortisol in the bloodstream. High levels of this stress hormone correlate with high blood pressure as well as inflammation and increased risk of cardiovascular disease.

Following a steam bath and a shower, David met Mary Ann in the lobby and invited her to lunch, but she asked for a rain cheque. She had promised to pick up her daughter, Erika, from school at noon, so the two of them could play hooky. Mary Ann explained that she occasionally needed to take a break from her hectic schedule. Either alone or with one of her two children she would take a day or a half a day off. Sometimes she would go to a movie; otherwise she would simply go for walk in a park or the countryside, taking time to smell the flowers and to lie on her back and gaze at the clouds.

*Cool,* thought David, *Habit 4 in action!*

"Before you go," David said, "Have you got any sage advice for quitting smoking? I know it's going to kill me, and I have read a few books and pamphlets but I'm afraid to quit."

"Why afraid?" asked Mary Ann.

"I guess I'm not looking forward to the withdrawal symptoms, the agitation, and the weight gain. Frankly, cigarettes have always been there for me in times of stress. This may sound stupid, but my cigarette is kind of my best friend … has been for over twenty-five years."

"I can understand that, David," she replied. "Having been a smoker for many years myself, I know exactly how you feel. While I was going through my divorce I remember lighting up a cigarette and experiencing a very familiar feeling of comfort. Logically, I knew that the cigarette was a false friend, as it cost me a lot of money, and like you, I knew it was destroying my health. But I could not think of anything to replace the unconditional, non-judging, acceptance and comfort I was getting from my addiction."

"So what did you do?" asked David.

"I knew I could not do it on my own, so I simply gave the problem over to God. I prayed that God would remove my fear of quitting and help me overcome any barriers that stood in my way. Four days later—on a sunny Sunday morning—I had made brunch for a few friends and realized I had not had a cigarette all morning. I reflexively lit a cigarette and had a puff, but it did not taste familiar, nor did it make me feel relaxed. The cigarette felt strange in my hand; I did not know how to hold it. I had held a cigarette between my index and middle fingers of my left hand for over twenty years, but suddenly it felt awkward. I tried my right hand—that was worse. I tried holding it like a joint—between my index finger and thumb of my left hand, then my right, but it felt like I was looking at someone else's hand holding the cigarette. I did not even remember my prayer of four days earlier until later, but I remember feeling puzzled and butting the cigarette out."

"One of my friends who had stayed behind after brunch to help me clean up, asked why I was not smoking. I told her that I had quit that morning. She said, 'Right, for how many hours, Mary Ann?'"

"But that was it." Mary Ann smiled with a wave of her hand. "I never smoked again. That was almost four years ago, and I know I will never smoke again. The strange thing is, I don't even miss it, and it is hard to think of myself as ever having smoked in the first place. I did not really gain weight either, as I made a conscious effort to go to the gym four times a week. I can't explain it, and have not told a lot of people this story, but you asked, so now you know. Got to go … can't keep Erika waiting!"

Feeling revived by his yoga practice and inspired by his conversation with Mary Ann, David returned to his apartment and picked up the now-familiar booklet he had found in the taxi. His heart attack was beginning to seem like a long time ago.

*No man is an island, entire of itself; every man is a piece of the continent.*

**John Donne** (c.1572–1631), British author

## HABIT FIVE: SOCIAL CONNECTEDNESS

On the roller coaster of life, the passengers affect each other; people are nourished by other people.

One of the important features that distinguish humans from other creatures is that we are social animals. We are designed to live in packs or tribes. We depend on each other; we are interdependent members of families and communities, even while we function independently.

We cannot live a full life in isolation from others; indeed, interacting with others and for others is an important determinant of individual and societal health. The group is greater than the sum of its parts. Certain communities have a high degree of social capital and have been used as an example of the beneficial effect of the "clan."

The town of Roseto in eastern Pennsylvania was a small homogeneous community where most of the inhabitants emigrated from the same Italian village in the late nineteenth century. It was noted that the men in this town had a radically lower rate of heart disease than their peers across the country and even in neighbouring communities. When this phenomenon was carefully studied, it turned out that the difference was not due to diet, nor exercise, nor genetic make-up. Rather, this particular community was very connected and egalitarian: there were many three generation families living under one roof and the elders commanded respect; residents knew their neighbours and frequently stopped to chat; they cooked for each other and cared for each other; most residents belonged to one or more of the many service clubs and civic organizations; they worshipped together at the same church and there were no demonstrable differences between those who were affluent and those who were less successful. In short, the people of Roseto thrived because of the high degree of social connections that flourished in their close-knit town and this translated into a lower mortality rate! The "Roseto Effect" has since been used as an example of the benefit of the Clan or social networking.[43]

"Hell" has sometimes been defined as being in isolation for eternity. While most of us would enjoy a few hours or even a day or two of peaceful solitude it would be unbearable to be alone for long periods of time. Imagine having no one to talk to, interact with, care for and love, nobody to sing and dance and travel with, no one to play sports with, compete with, bounce ideas off, no family dinners, no social gatherings or parties, no one to laugh or cry with, and nobody to impress or share your life with. Even prisoners in solitary confinement interact with guards and occasionally with other prisoners—and their sentence is not forever. We know the terrible pain and loneliness after a separation or bereavement, or even how much we miss friends and loved ones when we travel. Some people go through intense withdrawal if the Internet is down or they can't check e-mails or Facebook for a few days. Imagine being alone—forever. Clearly, we *need* to be with others; our personal survival and the sustainability of our society depend on it.

---

[43] Gladwell, Malcolm, 2008, The Roseto Mystery, *Introduction to Outliers,* Little, Brown and Company, New York, page 9

Social capital in a community is a concept that can be measured by assessing membership in voluntary groups and organizations such as service groups, clubs, and belonging to churches. It is exemplified by voter participation, getting together with friends and neighbours for sports, movies, dinners, bowling, and other social events.

Diminished social capital can occur because of various factors including longer commute times, resulting in the average North American spending twice as much time behind the wheel of their car than they do with their children. More time in front of television and computer screens, as well as crime and fear of violent crimes keeps citizens behind their automatic garage doors and in their gated communities.

Communities in which there is high social capital enjoy many benefits. These include greater attendance in post-secondary education, lower crime rates and violence, less poverty and also improved health outcomes.[44] It is interesting that different neighbourhoods even in the same city are more socially connected than others, resulting in a higher quality of life in terms of happiness, safety, income, and even health and life expectancy for the residents who live there.

Individuals, too, require a social connection to thrive. Being disconnected from family, friends, and community leads to isolation, loneliness, impaired immune function, and illness. As such, the altruistic deeds done by an

---

[44] Putnam, Robert, 2000, *Bowling Alone: The Collapse and Revival of American Community*, Simon & Shuster.
Dr. Putnam is a political scientist and professor of public policy at Harvard University.

individual for someone else benefit not only the recipient, but also the giver, and society at large. One's personal success, then, can be measured more appropriately by how much one gives rather than how much one possesses. Human beings are social animals, and we need to recognize and honour our interconnectedness. Unless we experience connection to others in a meaningful way, we risk developing spiritual, mental, and certainly physical illness.

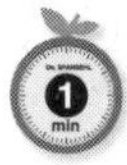

**One minute message**

A basic human need is for us to be in *social groups*. The connection between various people forms the fabric of a society. The more intense and diverse those relationships are, the stronger that *society* or *community* becomes.

*Give* of your time and resources to improve your community, which will ultimately be a benefit to yourself. Consider doing *volunteer work* at home or abroad, help out at your local hospital, join a faith-based group or service club, donate blood, organize neighbourhood get-togethers. Reconnect with former classmates, chat with colleagues, invite an old or a new friend home for dinner.

A good way in which to enhance social connections in our communities is by volunteering. There are plenty of opportunities to help out at hospitals, community centres, faith-based organizations, food banks, soup kitchens, homeless shelters, and sports events, to name just a few. This can be done in one's own community as well as abroad. It is important not to take our blessings for granted and to become more generous in giving of our time and resources. When we incorporate community service work into our regular routine, it yields benefits for both the giver and receiver of that effort. Remember to not limit kind words and deeds to strangers; helping out family and friends is equally important.

It's easy to become overwhelmed by the amount of suffering in our own countries as well as internationally. We cannot possibly help all the people and worthy causes that need us. Recognize that one can only do so much and that sometimes helping just one person can make a tremendous difference. Think about your interests and priorities and pick an activity deserving of your time and energy.

By interacting with others without expectation of getting anything in return, you acknowledge that we are all one and that the happiness of each is connected to the happiness of all. The more we put others' interests ahead of our own, the more we will experience the interconnectedness of all beings, and the healthier we will be.

Studies have shown that volunteering increases one's sense of connection to a community, gives meaning to life, instils a sense of well-being, and reduces stress by putting personal problems into perspective. It can also lower one's risk of coronary artery disease.

A culture of volunteerism is a critical part of a healthy and successful society. The opposite of being self-centred and self-absorbed, giving to someone or to a cause without expecting remuneration or acknowledgement is a characteristic of selflessness. As an additional benefit, much like blood donations being helpful for the donor as well as the recipient, the act of giving contributes to your personal development.

The improved sense of well-being that occurs when we give our time to others is particularly evident in older adults.[45] When a person says he or she is "high on life," that is an accurate and scientific assessment. Science has now discovered that volunteering and other pleasurable activities raise level of chemicals in the brain that make us feel good!

People who are "high on life" get a surge of serotonin from their daily activities. It is therefore essential to fill your day doing things that you are passionate about and make you feel that you are making a difference in the world. Being complimented for a job well done or receiving a sense of accomplishment from the successful completion of a challenge results in an increase in dopamine in our brains. This is a neurotransmitter involved in satisfaction and craving. It stands to reason, then, that if we set our lives up for success by choosing to spend time in work that we enjoy and in situations and with people that we love, that we can live this "natural high." Conversely, if we are stuck in dead end jobs and trapped in a bad relationship, and the friends we choose bring us down, it is no wonder that we will not feel happy, content, and fulfilled as individuals.

---

[45] Morrow-Howell N., et.al., 2003, Effects of volunteering on the well-being of older adults, The Journals of Gerontology, Series B; the Journal of Gerontology: *Psychological Sciences and the Journal of Gerontology: Social Sciences.*, May;58(3):S137–45.

*You must give some time to your fellow men. Even if it's a little thing, do something for others—something for which you get no pay but the privilege of doing it.*

**Dr. Albert Schweitzer** (1875–1965) Alsatian physician, theologian and musician—winner of Nobel Peace Prize 1952, reflecting on why he decided to do medical missionary work in Africa

---

" Connection to others, to community, as well as to nature, is important to reduce the illnesses that stem from self-centredness. Depression, anxiety, fatigue, and loneliness may have their roots in disconnectedness. To improve health and happiness, strive to connect with nature through activities such as hiking, gardening and family picnics. Connecting with pets also has numerous health advantages. Having pets (especially of various species) in the home has been shown to lower the risk of childhood allergies. (The Hygiene Hypothesis states that a little dirt never hurt. Kids who grow up in a sterile environment have less robust immune systems than do those kids who grow up with other children and animals.) Having a dog is an effective and inexpensive way for adults to get exercise. In addition, the unconditional love, acceptance and loyalty of pets make them ideal confidants of children, adolescents, and adults alike. Having a family dog, for example, reduces the risk of a teenager becoming dependent on recreational drugs.

“Connect with friends and family by taking the time to foster relationships and staying in touch. Connect with a higher power that makes us part of a larger reality. Join a program to explore your faith, and even if you are of no particular faith, allow yourself to explore the possibility of a greater creative power that connects us and makes us whole.

Building our personal infrastructure, fostering lasting relationships, and giving freely of our resources; time, talents, and money will increase our own health and raise the social capital of our communities.

---

*Society is the total network of relations between human beings. The components of society are thus not human beings but relations between them. In a societal structure individuals are merely the foci in the network of relationships ....*

*A visible and palpable collection of people is not a society; it is a crowd. A crowd, unlike a society, can be assembled, dispersed, photographed, and massacred.*

**Arnold Toynbee** (1852–1883) from “A Study of History”

---

David returned to Dr. Osler's office for a follow-up visit but was told that his doctor was running about an hour behind. Dr. Osler had a booking policy called "Advanced Access" in his office in which he tried to see most of the patients when they needed to be seen. He was therefore able to see a majority of patients that called for an appointment within one to two days. He tried to keep the appointments efficient and succinct as his staff booked him only ten minutes for a routine appointment. This included the time required to look up test results, print prescriptions, make referrals, and record his encounter in the Electronic Medical Record on his computer system.

That day, the wheels had fallen off the cart, however, as there were unforeseen delays on his hospital rounds in the morning, followed by a rash of urgent phone calls when he had gotten to his office, more people added on to his schedule than he had time to see, and problems that were too complex to deal with in the allotted time.[46]

David sat down beside an anxious-looking man in his early forties. He struck up a conversation with Kevin Phillips, who apologized that his jacket still smelled of cigarette

---

[46] Primary Care Renewal. Historically, Canadian physicians were compensated on a fee-for-service basis which sometimes resulted in a large number of patients being seen as quickly as possible. Physicians often felt rushed and complex patients may not have gotten the time or care they needed. Also, new grads who chose family practice as a specialty were more likely to work in a high volume walk-in clinic rather than sign up for full–service family practice, where they would need to attend hospital patients, see complicated patients, visit patients at home and be on call—often with less income than their colleagues who work at a clinic.

Volume limits were introduced and in 2007, the British Columbia Medical Association partnered with the Ministry of Health and the regional Health Authorities to create the *Practice Support Program*. This ambitious initiative included strategies and financial incentives designed to revitalize Family Practice; to make it possible to look after chronically ill patients more effectively, reduce hospitalizations, and improve long-term health outcomes for patients while providing appropriate compensation for complex medical conditions.

In Canada, the United States, and other counties, Primary Care Renewal has the Triple Aim to provide better access and medical care for individuals, better health for populations, and lower per capita costs. At the same time, an improved primary care system will allow family doctors to practice longer and attract more medical school graduates into family practice, in order to allow most citizens to have a family doctor and to reach the goals of improved health care.

smoke although he had quit three days beforehand. Kevin shared that he had suffered a heart attack and had a stent placed in one of his coronary arteries. Kevin was worried that he may have another heart attack, and that he may not be able to return to work, and that he may not see his two school-aged kids grow up. David realized with a surge of empathy that he was not the only forty-something person who had problems. Although the two patients were from different walks of life—Kevin was a maintenance manager at a suburban hospital—David saw that they had quite a bit in common. As best he could, he quietly encouraged Kevin that by quitting smoking he was taking a great first step in improving his health.

After Kevin had gone in to see Osler, David resumed reading his booklet that he had brought with him.

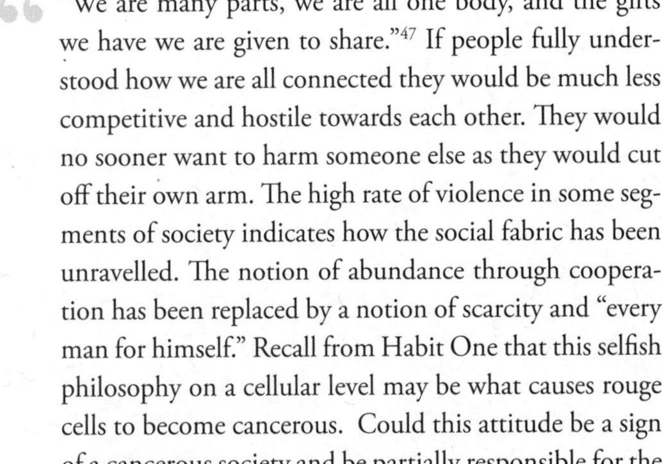

"We are many parts, we are all one body, and the gifts we have we are given to share."[47] If people fully understood how we are all connected they would be much less competitive and hostile towards each other. They would no sooner want to harm someone else as they would cut off their own arm. The high rate of violence in some segments of society indicates how the social fabric has been unravelled. The notion of abundance through cooperation has been replaced by a notion of scarcity and "every man for himself." Recall from Habit One that this selfish philosophy on a cellular level may be what causes rouge cells to become cancerous. Could this attitude be a sign of a cancerous society and be partially responsible for the sharp increase in cancer in the last one hundred years?

---

[47] Haugen, Marty, 1980, *We Are Many Parts*; a song of praise.

David remembered Osler asking him a few questions about friends and his social connections. This began to make sense as he read that men with a large circle of friends were almost half as likely to develop heart disease compared to men who had little social contact or support. Both casual friendships and deeper, more supportive relationships appeared to be protective of heart health.[48]

When it came time for his own appointment with Dr. Osler, David felt confident that he was on the right track. He would start his cardiac rehab program two days later. Osler advised him to use a nicotine inhaler when he had the urge to smoke. David had managed to cut back to less than half the amount he previously smoked, but was not ready to give up completely. However, now that he had seen that both Mary Ann and Kevin could quit, he figured he had a shot. His competitive streak was as strong as ever.

Osler found that these moments of motivation offered the ideal window of opportunity for making lasting changes in behaviour. It is always tempting for physicians to act like authority figures and sternly tell patients that they are too fat, they smoke too much, don't exercise enough—and if they don't change their evil ways, it will surely lead to an early grave. Interestingly, playing the power card with the white coat and stethoscope occasionally motivates (scares) some people. But it usually does not last, and as patients are

---

[48] Rosengren A,, et.al., 2004, Coronary disease in relation to social support and social class in Swedish men. A fifteen-year follow-up in the study of men born in 1933, *Department of Medicine*, Sahlgrenska University Hospital/Ostra, SE–416 85 Goteborg, Sweden. *European Heart Journal*, Jan;25(1):56–63. In this prospective study of men, two dimensions of low social support—low social integration and low emotional attachment—were found to be predictive of coronary morbidity, independently of other risk factors.

often ashamed to present to the doctor without having made the requested changes, they may stop coming altogether. So this paternalistic paradigm is considered "old school." What Osler preferred was a partnership with his patients. He would try to help them reach their own goals—not his.

That afternoon Dr. Osler encouraged David to "open your heart." He meant this figuratively as well as literally. By following a healthy lifestyle and taking his meds, David could open up his coronary arteries and reduce the risk of further blockages. "Cardiologist Dr. Dean Ornish has shown that lifestyle changes alone can reverse heart disease. His program includes a low-fat diet, regular exercise and relaxation, and perhaps most importantly, sessions with a psychologist to discuss life stressors and how we deal with them.[49] By being open and honest with friends or counsellors—that is by opening our hearts—we can deal with stressors more effectively and reduce our risk of heart disease," summed up Osler.

---

[49] Ornish, 1990, *Dr. Dean Ornish's Program For Reversing Heart Disease*, Ivy Books, New York, Published by Ballantine Books. Dr. Ornish measured the amount of blockage in coronary arteries before and after his lifestyle program and was able to demonstrate improvement without medications or surgery.

*It is man's social nature which distinguishes him from the brute creation. If it is his privilege to be independent, it is equally his duty to be inter-dependent. Only an arrogant man will claim to be independent of everybody else and be self-contained .... Man becomes great exactly in the degree in which he works for the welfare of his fellow-men.*

**Mahatma Gandhi** (1869–1948)

.....................................................................

Osler had asked David to come up with his "Top Ten Foods." David had enjoyed this exercise and put together the list based on the research he had done as well his own personal preferences. He indicated to Osler that this was not a definitive list, but his best attempt as of today, realizing that as he learned more, or his preferences changed, the list would change.

**Top ten foods:**

10. **Chocolate**. "The healthy part of chocolate is the cocoa; choose rich, dark chocolate, with a minimum of 70 percent cocoa. Avoid low-quality bars high in sugar and harmful oils," read David from his notes. "Cocoa contains heart-healthy and mood enhancing phytochemicals and antioxidants particularly compounds called polyphenols or flavanols, so named as they give colour and flavour to foods." "Agreed," replied Osler. "These are also found in wine and tea as well as deeply-pigmented fruits and vegetables. They have been shown to inhibit platelet

aggregation and inhibit oxidation of LDL, the bad form of cholesterol. Oxidized cholesterol increases the risk of heart attacks and strokes. Flavanols relax blood vessels and stimulate glucose absorption. In this way, dark chocolate helps to lower blood pressure and improve insulin sensitivity.[50] White chocolate would have no effect and milk chocolate may have a modest effect. Cocoa has also been shown to improve the flexibility of blood vessels in particular by improving the inner lining of arteries—something called endothelial function." Seeing that David was interested in the chemicals in chocolate, Osler continued. "Cocoa also contains *theobromine*, a compound similar to caffeine and an asthma drug called theophylline. This substance can open bronchial airways, elevate the mood and is actually addictive! Other mood-altering substances found in cocoa include *phenethylamine*, a neuro-chemical associated with sexual arousal that is released in the brain when people fall in love. Another is *anandamide*, which binds to same receptors as cannabinoids (the active ingredient in marijuana) producing feelings of euphoria. Chocolate also boosts brain levels of serotonin, similar to many antidepressant medications."

"I'm impressed," said David, "No wonder I crave the stuff."

"There is a caution or two," replied Osler. "A modest one-to two-ounce serving a few times a week will suffice. My preference is to choose organic fair trade products that are now readily available."

---

[50] Grassi, D., et.al., 2005, Short-term administration of dark chocolate is followed by a significant increase in insulin sensitivity and a decrease in blood pressure in healthy persons., *American Journal of Clinical Nutrition*, Vol. 81, No. 3, 611–614, March

9. **Red wine**. "I do enjoy a glass or two with dinner," said David. "And my work involves a lot of eating out." Dr. Osler looked thoughtful. "As alcohol is addictive and a neurotoxin, it should only be consumed in moderation, and only by individuals who are not at risk of addiction. However, for those who take pleasure in an occasional drink, there is a lot to be said for consuming the fruit of the vine. There are benefits reported with both white and red wine consumption. Red wine, in particular contains resveratrol, a potent antioxidant." "*Proanthocyanidins*, a family of flavonoids found in wine, may inhibit platelet aggregation. Small amounts of alcohol consumed regularly may also raise HDL levels. Epidemiological—that is population based—studies indicate that those who consume a moderate amount of alcohol have better health outcomes than those who drink a lot (no surprise), but also compared to those who abstain from alcohol altogether. It is not clear whether there are any confounding variables that would make this so, or if there is indeed benefit from the wine. On balance, if you enjoy wine, you should not be discouraged from consuming one to two glasses two to three times a week."

8. **Wild salmon**. "I love salmon," said David. "And now I know that in addition to providing good protein, oily fish are also the best source of the healthy omega-3 fats known as DHA and EPA, which have been shown to improve cholesterol levels, concentration, memory, and mood, and reduce the risk of heart disease, cancer, arthritis, and other inflammatory conditions." He said glancing at his notes again.

"That's right," said Osler. "Plant sources of omega-3 fatty acids—ALA (alpha linolenic acid)—can be converted to the longer-chain fatty acids found in fish that humans require, so that fish is not essential in the diet. However, the conversion to the long-chain fatty acids is inefficient and is influenced by other foods. Therefore, it's much easier to get optimal amounts of the important fatty acids by including oily fish in the diet."
"Large fish have been found to be contaminated with mercury, and concerns have been raised over farmed salmon carrying lice that may be harmful to wild salmon and their ecosystems, so it is important to know the source of any fish you consume. I also enjoy sardines as these small fish are very nutritious and uncontaminated. Incidentally, fish-oil supplements are distilled and therefore free of harmful heavy metals."

7. **Green tea**. "Besides being known as a healthy beverage, I have actually acquired a taste for the subtle flavour of a good green tea." David continued, "I read that all tea leaves come from same plant: *Camellia sinensis*. Green tea is produced by only drying the leaves, for oolong tea, the leaves are partially fermented, and black tea is more fermented to intensify the flavour. White tea is made from the air-dried tips of tea plants. Both green and black teas have been credited with heart-protecting and cancer-inhibiting powers, but fermentation changes some polyphenols, so green tea is the preferred choice."
"True," said Osler. "Researchers speculate that the antioxidant polyphenols (or catechins) in tea may inhibit certain mechanisms that promote cancer growth,

especially in the esophagus, stomach, colon, breast, and prostate. Polyphenols (especially one known as EGCG found in green tea) can relax blood vessels and thereby help control blood pressure. The anti-inflammatory and free-radical scavenging properties of green tea have also been credited for keeping the mind sharper and reducing neurodegenerative conditions such as Alzheimer's and Parkinson's disease. In addition, green tea can sooth and protect skin (used topically as well as internally), and it speeds up your body's metabolism, helping to control weight. But you may have to drink several cups per day to produce a beneficial effect.[51] This is a great list, David—what have you chosen next?" Doctor Osler asked.

6. **Walnuts** and other nuts. "I was surprised to read about the health benefits of nuts," said David, "in particular for diabetics and those with high cholesterol." "Yes, there've been many studies," said Osler. "An analysis of multiple clinical food trials showed that eating about seven walnuts a day lowered the LDL (bad) cho-

---

[51] Basu A., Lucas E.A., 2007, Mechanisms and effects of green tea on cardiovascular health, *Nutrition Review* 65:361–75.

[52] Banel, D.K., Hu, FB, 2009, Effects of walnut consumption on blood lipids and other cardiovascular risk factors: a meta-analysis and systematic review, *American Journal of Clinical Nutrition*, vol. 90 no. 1 56-63. Consumption of a walnut-rich diet leads to significant improvements in total and low-density lipoprotein cholesterol.
Abbey, M., Noakes, M., Belling, G.B., Nestel, P.J., 1994, Partial replacement of saturated fatty acids with almonds or walnuts lowers total plasma cholesterol and low-density-lipoprotein cholesterol. *American Journal of Clinical Nutrition*, Vol. 59, 995-999.

[53] Anderson, J.W., 2003, Diet May Lower Cholesterol as Much as Statins, *Journal of the American Medical Association*, 290:502–510, 531–533.

lesterol seven percent.[52] Another study revealed that almonds are 'as effective as statins' in lowering LDL.[53] Almonds contain mostly monounsaturated fats and are high in trace minerals such as magnesium, zinc, selenium, and they are also high in fibre. Most nuts and grains have a beneficial effect on lipids and also seem to relax and dilate blood vessels. Walnuts, in particular, are high in the heart-healthy omega-3 fatty acid, ALA. The Nurses' Health Study in Boston monitored 86,000 nurses; those who ate five ounces of nuts per week had one-third fewer heart attacks than those who ate the fewest nuts." "They are high in fat and calories, though," David countered. "Correct," his doctor replied, "but mixed, unsalted, raw, or dry-roasted nuts have benefits for both blood glucose control and blood lipids and may be used as part of a strategy to improve health without weight gain."

5. **Broccoli.** "Turns out that Mom was right," said David. "Broccoli is a member of the cabbage family, and these are all very good for you. Broccoli sprouts are even better, apparently, although I don't think I've eaten them." Osler nodded. "Sulphoraphanes were recently shown to inhibit Helicobacter pylori, the bug that causes ulcers; they also arm your body to fight other infections. Along with pulses and other cruciferous vegetables, chemical substances in broccoli have been shown to reduce breast, colon, and lung cancer. All green vegetables are also good source of B vitamins such as folic acid, as well as fibre."

4. **Blueberries**. "This is one food everyone in our family agrees on," said David. "But until this week, I had no idea how good they are for you." Osler smiled. "*Anthocyanidins*, the pigments that give blueberries their colour and flavour have been shown to reduce macular degeneration and memory loss. Similar compounds called *proanthocyanidins* are found in blueberries, cranberries, and acai berries. These antioxidants along with a carbohydrate called d-mannose, also found in berries, seem to be helpful in treating and preventing urinary tract infections by reducing the ability of bacteria such as E. coli to adhere to the bladder wall. The U.S. Department of Agriculture Human Nutrition Center on Aging at Tufts University in Boston, compared forty different types of fruits and vegetables in an antioxidant contest—and blueberries took first place."

3. **Flax seeds.** "I knew that flax was used to make linen and linseed oil, but I never knew they could be eaten until I did some reading on miracle foods! They should be ground, preferably organically grown, and stored in glass in the fridge or freezer," said David, again consulting his notes. "Yes," said Osler. "Flax is rich in soluble and insoluble fibre, lignans, and alpha linolenic acid (an essential omega-3 fatty acid), making it valuable in the battle against heart disease, as well as cancers of the prostate and breast, and is a great way to clean the intestinal tract."

2. **Soy and other legumes**. "I know that beans and lentils are a great source of vegetable protein," said David, "and that they have been a staple food in many

cultures as they are inexpensive and nutritious." Osler nodded. "Indeed, pulses—or legumes—are a good source of plant-based protein as well as fibre, vitamins, and minerals. There were some concerns raised over the phytoestrogens in soy beans, as they stimulate estrogen receptors. Estrogens may cause breast cancer, or an abnormal growth of the lining of the uterus. However, the plant estrogens are far weaker than human hormones and therefore mostly block estrogen receptors. Japanese women who eat a traditional high soy diet have one-fifth the rate of breast cancer as North American women do. You've done your homework well, David", Doctor Osler complimented his patient, "I'm curious what you have chosen to top your list."

1. **Pure water.** "The elixir of life has to be number one!" enthused David. "Humans consist of approximately 65 percent water, so this is the most essential nutrient for our bodies. Or so I'm told." "Yes, water hydrates us, aids with digestion and metabolism, circulates nutrients (through blood) and flushes impurities out of our bodies through sweat, urine, and feces," replied Osler. "Water helps control body temperature and cushions the joints. By contrast, lack of water is thought to be the primary cause of daytime fatigue." "A mere two percent drop in body water can trigger fuzzy short-term memory, trouble with basic math, and difficulty focusing. Drinking approximately two litres of clear fluids (filtered tap water and green tea) each day has been shown to reduce hunger pangs, ease back and joint pains, improve brain function, and diminish the risk of colon, breast, and bladder cancer. Thirst is a signal that you are

already one to two percent dehydrated. Generally, if you drink water with and between meals and with increased activities, you will be getting enough. The other 'gold standard' of ensuring enough water intake is by monitoring your urine. If you are voiding less than four times a day you may not be drinking enough. The urine should be pale yellow in colour. If it is dark and concentrated you may be mildly dehydrated. Note that B-vitamins can turn the urine a bright yellow colour."

Osler then asked David what he thought about including meats. "I do enjoy a good steak," said David. "But in general I wonder whether meat is healthy enough to include in my top ten foods. Osler mentioned that meats not produced in factory farms are higher in Omega 3s and are less likely to contain hormones and antibiotics. They could therefore be considered part of a healthy diet, "My father used to take me along on hunting trips when I still lived at home. The wide variety of game and fowl that we shot were an important part of our family's nutrition."

"My grandfather, who lived a long and healthy life, used to hunt as well and he often washed down his venison with wine. We discussed wine earlier but I'm not clear on why modest amounts of alcohol are related to better health." asked David.

"Well, alcohol itself kills brain cells so the biological plausibility of it being good for us is not high. Furthermore, the antioxidants found in wine are also found in fruit juices—which have not been found to be as beneficial. So I do not think that resveritrol alone, or other antioxidants account for the protective effect of wine. I also don't believe in the French Paradox."

The *French Paradox* was an observation that French people suffered a lower incidence of coronary heart disease than North Americans and even other Europeans, despite having a diet relatively rich in saturated fats. This was wishfully attributed to resulting from the higher consumption of red wine in that country. Others felt it may be due to lower levels of refined carbohydrates being consumed, however, it may simply have been based on inaccurate statistics.

"In my opinion," continued Dr. Osler, "better health outcomes are related to wine consumption because the alcohol acts as a stress reliever. If, after a hectic day, one sits down with some good company and good wine (or even a beer or a cocktail) it certainly has a relaxing effect. If someone does not have a tendency towards addiction, I do not dissuade my patients from enjoying an occasional fermented beverage."

"What about spices?" asked David. "I couldn't figure out where to put them on my Top Ten list," said David. "From what I've read, it's a good idea to eat garlic and turmeric on a daily basis, but I could not really fit them in as *foods*."

"Yes, I too am impressed with the benefits of turmeric, and its active component, curcumin, said Osler. "There are known anti-inflammatory effects, which may explain the cardiovascular benefits as well as its anti-cancer role. It may also partly explain why people living in India have a lower incidence of dementia than those of us in the West."

"I wish I'd known some of these facts a long time ago," said David. I'm stunned by all the ways that food directly influences our health."

Osler suggested that David strive for a new model of eating. "The North American diet typically contains slow proteins and fast carbs: it is full of heavy, slowly-digested meats and 'white foods' such as white flour, white sugar, white rice, mashed potatoes, and overcooked pasta," he continued. "Given our often sedentary lives, we need more legumes and fish, and also whey protein powder in fruit shakes. Focus as well on whole foods—nuts, seeds, whole grains, and vegetables. The combination of foods will result in a 'fast protein, slow carbohydrate' diet. This high-fibre diet will provide sustained energy and satiety for many hours without a spike in the blood sugar and insulin levels," he concluded.

"It's interesting to hear you say that", said David, "as it is similar to what the trainer at the gym advised me. He reminded me to hydrate well before and after workout and also recommended whole grains and other complex carbs prior to the workout for fuel and then protein in the golden hour after a work-out to strengthen and repair my muscles."

Osler asked David to see him again in two weeks to review how he was doing and develop an exercise program.

David caught a cab back home. While he missed driving his own car, he quite liked having a driver take him door to door, without having to stress about traffic and worry about finding parking. Also, when he added up the cost of gas, parking, insurance, licensing, and the car payments, he realized that he was much further ahead taking the taxi.

Back in his apartment, David enjoyed a smoked salmon on rye sandwich along with a small salad. After cleaning up, he made himself a cup of Yerba Mate, a traditional tea-like drink popular in South America, where it is valued as a healing beverage. David found it to be invigorating, and when he read that it stimulates the immune system, he had decided to give it a try. He particularly enjoyed mixing it with jasmine green tea. David sat down at his desk, answered a few e-mails, and then called Joanna Lee from the law firm to discuss some of his files that she was working on. It was a bit shocking when it occurred to him that this was a Friday, and yet he felt none of the tiredness that he usually did at the end of his work week. How would it be when he returned to the firm full time?

On the following morning, David cycled to the sports field to watch Adam's soccer game. While the Orcas played, David walked up and down the side lines with the coach, Justin Rose, whose son Mathias spent a lot of time with Adam kicking the soccer ball around or just hanging out. David remembered that he had had many friends as a kid and thought about how easy it was to talk about whatever was on his mind. His closest friends had been Andrew and Scott. The three of them had stuck together through thick and thin. No bullies could touch them as they had strength in numbers. They had shared joys and adventures as well as hardships—whether about teachers, parents, or other kids. Without being aware of it they had lived the Chinese philosophy that *shared joy is double joy and shared sorrow is half sorrow.*

When he had attended university, he again had two close friends, Berny and Stan, with whom he had shared some great adventures—skiing and hiking trips and a six- month journey through Europe following their graduation. After college, they had all settled in different cities, and eventually had drifted apart.

David realized that he really did not have any close friends anymore. He knew many people, enjoyed socializing, and still got together with his buddies from law school for drinks, but he did not have a confidante with whom he could share his thoughts, ideas, and fears. Jessica had filled that role. His friendships had become more superficial—kind of like flipping through TV channels with the remote control—pausing to watch a while, but then moving on when he lost interest. He also did not want to come across as weak by burdening his acquaintances with his problems, so he generally kept his emotions to himself.

When the game was over and they were packing up, David felt compelled to say, "On your way home, pick up some flowers for your wife and tell her how much you love her."

Justin replied, "You miss Jessica very much, don't you?"

"I can't begin to explain to you how much I'm still grieving the loss of our relationship. This hurts me far more than my heart attack did, and will take me longer to get over. I can't help but wonder if the strain in our relationship was somehow related to why I had my heart attack."

"Things are so different now. I love my children very much, and they love me and know that I will do everything I can to be a good father to them, but they prefer to spend time with their mother, because it's more fun. Until I wound up in hospital, I was the one who still had to go to work each day to make a living to support two households. On days when I had the kids I rushed home at six, made or picked up dinner, helped them with their homework, and put them to bed. They came home from school to an empty apartment, let themselves in with the key and waited for me. I still needed to keep the place clean, do laundry, buy groceries, and do all the things that their mother used to do and that I took for granted. On days they are with their mother, things are as they always have been. When they come home, either

Jessica or her parents are waiting for them with a smile and a home-cooked meal, and then they spend an enjoyable evening together. There's no way that I can compete with that, and the kids know it."

"In any relationship, there are things that you absolutely love about your partner and there are some things that may be more challenging. When you love each other, the positive attributes in the relationship sustain it. The negative things you either learn to live with, or you work on them together. I'm not sure that Jessica ever really loved me. So the challenges in our relationship became insurmountable obstacles for her. I don't know whether there was ever a spiritual bond between us … a reason greater than ourselves to stay together. I still love Jessica, and I always will. I admire her sense of humour, her intelligence, and her beauty. I doubt that I'll ever find anybody like her. Sorry, Justin, I did not mean to unload this on you."

"David, I'm happy to talk to you any time you like. Why don't you bring Adam by to play with Mathias sometime soon, and we'll have a chance to catch up," suggested Justin.

David agreed and thanked Justin for his kindness. He had never found it easy to open up to his peers and was not sure that he would feel comfortable doing so again anytime soon. In particular now, that he was single, he felt the need to foster some stronger friendships.[54]

As it was a warm day, David took the long way home, soaking up the sun during his bike ride along False Creek. Instead of feeling sorry for himself when he got to his

---

[54] Bentall, David, 2004, *The Company You Keep: The Transforming Power of Male Friendship.* Augsberg Books, Minneapolis.

apartment, he had a shower and tried a recipe from his new found booklet. It was simple, yet matched the healthy criteria that he and Osler had talked about. "I never imagined I'd be whipping up fruit smoothies in my blender," he said out loud. "But here I go."

**Antioxidant Power Smoothy**

2–4 Tbsp. whey protein isolate (with greens powder)
2 Tbsp. essential fatty acids oil (omega 3 and 6)
1 cup yogurt or kefir
2 cups seasonal fruits and berries (fresh or frozen)
1 cup frozen kale (freezing greens makes them easier to blend smoothly)
2 Tbsp. ground almonds
1 Tbsp. each of ground flax, hemp hearts, and chia seeds
1 Tbsp. of fresh ginger
½ tsp. turmeric
½ tsp. cinnamon
Milk or soy milk (or water) and ice as required.

# CHAPTER 7

*It is only with the heart that one can see rightly; what is essential is invisible to the eye.*

—from The Little Prince —
**Antoine de Saint-Exupery**
(1900–1944), French writer and aviator

"You're looking chipper today, David," commented Osler.

David indicated that he was walking and cycling more—he had biked to his appointment—and was attending the Peninsula Club three to four times a week.

Dr. Osler mentioned a study he had recently read in a medical journal. Over a year, researchers at the University of Leipzig in Germany had conducted a randomized trial comparing the effects of angioplasty (opening a narrowed coronary artery with a balloon catheter and leaving a stent in place to hold it open) versus a regular exercise program in patients with coronary artery disease. Participants in the exercise group were conditioned in hospital on an exercise bike for ten minutes, six times a day, for two weeks. On discharge, they continued an aerobic workout on the bike for twenty minutes a day plus a sixty-minute group training session once a week.

Not surprisingly, the exercise group was found to have improved oxygen uptake and exercise tolerance. But they were also found to have less progression of the coronary artery plaque and a higher cardiac event-free survival compared to the group that had the angioplasty. So while the angioplasty group had the narrowing in their coronary arteries opened, the exercise group reaped benefits in their entire cardiovascular systems. In addition, the exercise treatment was significantly less expensive than the intervention group,

---

[55] Hambrecht, Rainer, et al., 2004, Percutaneous Coronary Angioplasty Compared With Exercise Training in Patients With Stable Coronary Artery Disease: A Randomized Trial. *Circulation*, Vol. 109 (No.11) Mar 23, p.1371–1378.

as fewer hospitalizations and procedures were needed.[55]

"Exercise also has spin-off benefits such as an overall improved level of fitness and strength, improved posture and confidence, better sleep and satisfaction," added Osler. "And as you age, the physical benefits are huge, but the cognitive benefits may be even more dramatic. Physical exercise is one of the few stimuli that results in the formation of new neurons (neurogenesis) in adults. Continued learning and positive attitude are factors that promote existing neurons taking on new functions (neuroplasticity). Some groundbreaking research done on aging and the mind came from The Nun Study."[56]

David's curiosity was piqued. "What happened there?" Osler sat back in his chair. It was one of those exceedingly rare days when he wasn't rushed off his feet. And there was nothing he liked to do more than to teach and inspire his patients.

"The Nun Study is an ongoing research project done by epidemiologist Dr. David Snowdon. It's one of the largest studies on Alzheimer's disease (AD). It involves 678 nuns ranging in age from seventy to over one hundred who live in convents of the School Sisters of Notre Dame, Minnesota. The study involves interviews, blood tests, MRI studies, and—for many of the nuns who consented—an autopsy. By analyzing autobiographies the nuns wrote as young women entering the convents, researchers were able to predict with nearly 90 percent certainty which nuns would develop Alzheimer's dementia sixty years later. Isn't that remarkable?"

---

[56] Snowdon, David, 2001 *Aging With Grace, What the Nun Study Teaches Us About Leading Longer Healthier and More Meaningful Lives.* Bantam

Dr. Osler asked.

David nodded.

"However, some surprising lessons were learned by studying the outliers as well. It turns out that a small number of the nuns who wrote very positive and diverse autobiographies (that would predict protection from AD) and showed no outward manifestations of the disease, in fact had advanced changes of AD noted on autopsy. It would appear that even for people predisposed to developing dementia, exercise, continued learning, leadership, and a passionate commitment to work helped them to live longer, happier lives and remain cognitively intact."

That evening, after dinner, David turned to his "taxi book" as he thought of it.

*Nothing in life is more wonderful than faith—the one great moving force which we can neither weigh in the balance nor test in the crucible.*

**Sir William Osler** (1849–1919)

Canadian physician and professor of medicine at McGill University, Montreal, Quebec, then Johns Hopkins University, Baltimore, Maryland, then Oxford University, England

**HABIT SIX: SPIRITUAL AWARENESS**

There is more robust scientific evidence to support the role of prayer in healing than many other medical interventions! Therefore, it follows that to deny oneself the healing power of prayer would be as ill-advised as denying any other proven medical intervention.[57]

" Research has shown that people who report that they are spiritual also feel better about their health. An assessment of the health perceptions of older adults revealed that the people who reported being the most spiritual also tended to rate their health more highly as compared to people who did not consider themselves to be spiritual.[58]

Being spiritual can mean different things to different people. People may feel spiritual when they meditate or pray, when they contemplate the meaning of life, when they commune with nature, when they are in the company of inspirational people, when they read sacred or meaningful books, when they are moved by art or music, or when they attend worship services at their chosen religious institution. Connecting with our inner selves, then, helps to create balance and harmony in our lives and also improves how healthy we feel. In addition to strengthening spiritual connections, there is good scientific evidence that prayer and meditation reduce anxiety, depression and headaches, lower blood pressure and cholesterol, and improve quality of life as well as life span.

Spirituality and faith may seem nebulous and difficult to prove. This is not a habit that is easily explained, nor can objective recommendations be given as for diet, exercise, and sleep. In fact, we sometimes tell someone to "take it on faith" if there is no hard evidence, but the advice comes from a trusted source.

---

[57] Dossey, Larry, 1999, Reinventing Medicine—Beyond Mind-Body to a New Era of Healing, Harper San Francisco, and Healing Words: The Power of Prayer and the Practice of Medicine, 1993.

[58] Daaleman, T.P., et.al., 2004, Religion, spirituality, and health status in geriatric outpatients, *Annals of Family Medicine*; 2:49–53.

There have been countless arguments brought forward to prove—or disprove—the existence of God. A scientific basis for intelligent creation is that of creating order out of chaos. An external force is a mandatory prerequisite to establishing order from randomly occurring particles and events.

Therefore, the creation of a system as complex as our universe must have depended on some sort of manipulation by an external force. The chance of the universe having formed randomly or spontaneously is so small that the statistical probability would be incalculable.

If you found a watch on a beach, you would know that a watchmaker must have designed it. This complex and intricate device could not have formed by itself. A supreme creative force may be impossible to quantify, yet that does not mean that it does not exist. Fundamental truths and laws of nature, such as gravity, exist whether we believe in them or not.[59]

Many people believe that there is a divine creative force that is responsible for the world that we live in (and have a duty to protect). Many also believe that we are somehow accountable to this Higher Power, and that our lives here on earth are not all that there is. It is comforting to know that death may not be the end—but the beginning of a new life. Various world religions have a different understanding of what the hereafter may be like and what our *souls* or *spirits* are—and how they live on; yet there is a fundamental agreement that

---

[59] Dumouchel, E., 2010, Some of the ideas in this paragraph were extracted from: Use of brain leads many to belief in God, MC[2] (Journal of Mensa Canada Communications) Vol. 43 no.3, pg. 13.

when we leave this world we will enter another existence that we can't even imagine. While we can never experience this until we die—numerous near-death experiences and witnessing the passing of others gives us a tiny glimpse into what this may be like. In addition, there is compelling evidence of the truth and authenticity of the Bible.

Like love—which is hard to describe or prove to someone who has never experienced it—the profound joy and peace that can be found in faith is difficult to convey to non-believers. However, faith is about more than being happy; faith involves a personal relationship with our God. This relationship, like other important relationships requires communication. This dialogue is called prayer. Prayers may be spoken aloud in groups or by individuals, or they can be silent conversations and reflections in the stillness of our hearts. Faith is a journey we take that resonates with who we are and what we believe; it gives structure and framework to behaviour and meaning to our lives.

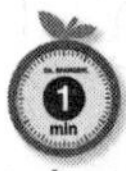

**One minute message**

Treat all people with *love* and *respect*—just as you would like to be treated.

Gather the *courage* to explore your own *faith* and our connection to a greater creative power by visiting a place of worship, pondering nature, meditating, wilderness hiking, or cloud and star gazing.

*Pray constantly: what breathing is for the body, prayer is for the soul.*

**St. Thomas Aquinas** (1225–1274) Italian priest, philosopher, and theologian (also attributed to St. Augustine of Hippo: 354–430)

David's grandfather had been a preacher who was very strict with his children. His son, David's father, had stopped attending church as soon as his dad had passed away. As a result, David had rarely attended church services; however, it was very important for his mother that David was married in church, and so he and Jessica had obliged her. He had not felt that a church wedding was necessary to seal his bond with Jessica, but his mom had felt that it somehow made their union more sacred and legitimate. David and Jessica agreed that it was a public celebration of their commitment to each other, as well as a festive occasion for family and friends to get together. After the wedding, church-going had played little or no role in their lives. David did not consider himself to be a "spiritual" being.

With the insights that *12 Habits* provided, David now felt that he was breaking some new ground in his recovery. The booklet had given him plenty of food for thought; he had never taken the time to explore his inner feelings and beliefs, so maybe this was the time to do so. He began reading again, wondering what other gems his taxi book had in store for him.

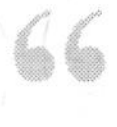

Forgiveness means giving up your resentment and bitterness. By not forgiving, you pay a significant negative price emotionally, mentally, and physically.

> Forgiveness applies equally to yourself as well as to others. The greatest benefactor of forgiveness is the forgiver, not necessarily the forgiven. Forgiveness does not mean you condone or accept what occurred; you are simply forgiving the person(s) for the act. Love the sinner, even while you hate the sin.

---

*Forgiveness is not an occasional act; it is a permanent attitude.*

**Martin Luther King, Jr.** (1929–1968) African American clergyman and civil rights activist.

---

David put down his book and thought for a while. He spent much of his time in court arguing for the defense that an alleged event couldn't be proven and in convincing a judge and jury that there was reasonable doubt. He didn't necessarily want his clients to be forgiven; he wanted to win his cases. In his personal life, however, David could see some use in separating the act from the actor—such as the idiot driver who had cut in front of his car a few days ago. Perhaps now was the time to see this person as another human being with his own stressors. Maybe David could also slow down and let go a bit himself.

> Positive *affirmations* and positive thinking can lead to the desired outcomes being manifested into your life. To affirm something is to declare strongly and publically that something is true. You can similarly affirm

intentions.
– *I choose to have a great day.*
– *I look forward to meeting with my boss.*
– *I'm sure I can make this sale.*
– *I know that I can reach my normal weight.*
– *I'm proud to be a non-smoker.*
– *My body is healthy and heals quickly.*
– *I can beat this cancer.*
– *I love my quiet home in the country.*

When you awake in the morning, set your intention for how you want the day to go and what you would like to accomplish. Sometimes by confidently and repeatedly articulating our intention, and clearly visualizing the desired outcome, it will become a self-fulfilling prophesy. The opposite is also true. If you believe that the new boss is going to be a jerk—he or she probably will be. If you fear that someone could not possibly be interested in you—they won't be. If you feel you could not possibly dunk a basketball—don't even try it. If you believe that you have no chance to get a better job—don't bother submitting an application. If you are convinced that you are condemned to a life of chronic pain and impaired functioning, then you may never feel better. If you see yourself as an out-of-shape and overweight sloth, that becomes your reality.

Affirmations are positive statements about how you

[60] Murphy, Jim, 2010. To learn more about how to use your mind to be successful in sports and business, read: *Inner Excellence—Achieve Extraordinary Business Success Through Mental Toughness.* New York: McGraw-Hill

would like to see yourself in the future, made as though they were true today.[60] You do not even need to believe your affirmation at first—if it were all true already, you would not need to keep affirming your intentions. You just need to *want* it to be true and make the affirmations part of your strategy to reach your goal. Like an actor, you need to convincingly behave *as if* your affirmation were true—and gradually, it can transform you.

Combine affirmations with belly breathing to create an effective mantra. For example, if you want to give up smoking but fear withdrawal and anxiety, you can practice deep breathing to feel the relaxation you get from smoking.

Try taking a slow breath in—like a drag on a cigarette—while you say, "I feel … " then exhale slowly while you say "calm and relaxed." Try four slow breaths, in through the nose and out through the mouth, first thing in the morning, and before you go to sleep. In addition, take four breaths throughout the day whenever you have the urge to smoke. You can even bring your hand to your mouth and inhale through your mouth as though you were puffing on a cigarette. You can say the mantra, "I feel … calm and relaxed" out loud or to yourself. The important thing is to make the affirmations an unequivocal statement of fact, no different than saying, "It is nice and sunny today" or "My name is John." Similarly, before attending an important meeting or prior to giving a speech, you can say, "I am … confident and articulate."

Try any affirmation you wish, breathing in to your belly and then out in a big sigh …

I feel … alert and energetic. (In the morning or when energy is waning in the afternoon.)

> I am ... healthy and strong.
> My body ... heals quickly.
> I am ... efficient and punctual.
> I am ... financially successful.
> I love ... my new job.
> I feel ... happy and content.
> I feel ... tremendous!
>
> So live each day on purpose—with clearly-articulated goals. Look for the good in people and maintain a positive outlook in times of uncertainly. Change is inevitable—and many times change may indeed be for the better.

The following day, David cycled down to the Peninsula Club for a spinning class. After his steam bath and shower he sat down at the juice bar, where he was pleased to bump into Mary Ann. She had just been in a yoga class and was starting her shift in a few hours, but was glad to have another opportunity to talk to David.

"I've been reading a bit about spirituality," said David, "I know there is a spiritual side of me that I would like to explore further, but I'm not sure that attending a church would bring me any closer to God."

Mary Ann paused before she answered. "Maybe—but don't just dismiss the importance of the Church. I see so many people in need in the course of my work," she began. "It's easy to forget that historically, the early Christians were committed to healing the sick, educating commoners, and feeding the hungry. In Biblical times, the sick were outcasts and were forced to live in the outskirts of town, shouting "unclean" to passers-by so they would not come close. The Church was responsible for some of the first hospitals, and even today religious orders continue to operate thousands of hospitals around the world and do a vast amount of medical mission work. Mother Teresa's Sisters of Charity come to mind. In addition, faith-based groups operate schools in nearly every community, and some of the most prestigious universities in the world were founded by the Jesuits or other religious orders. And don't forget the dozens of homeless shelters and soup kitchens in our city that are run by religious organizations. Personally, I'm able to do some volunteer work through my church to help others—and I get a lot of satisfaction from being in a spiritual community."

David had never really thought about religion in that way, but it was obviously an important part of Mary Ann's life. She radiated inner peace and confidence and encouraged David to join her at church the next Sunday.

"Thank you, Mary Ann," he replied, "I will certainly think about it." He left unsaid the fact that his Sunday mornings without the kids were usually spent catching up on work or watching sports on TV.

..........

On his next visit, David asked Dr. Osler whether he thought spirituality had a role in health. Osler said thoughtfully: "I have no doubt that a meaningful connection to a higher power is helpful, and I am aware of studies related to prayer and healing. But I don't feel it is my role as a doctor to explore a patient's spiritual beliefs or allow my own moral values to dictate the care I give."

"My primary job is to ensure that my patients receive timely and appropriate medical care regardless of where they are on life's journey," continued Osler. "However, I have observed that a patient's beliefs do influence their health decisions ... and outcomes."

.........................................................................

On his next trip to the Peninsula Club, David checked out a few of the recipe cards that were available at the juice bar. As he was committed to a healthier diet, he felt he should make more foods for himself so that he could select nutritious ingredients. He had tried the Vitality Muffins and thought he could tackle the directions.

**VITALITY MUFFINS**

2 cups flour
(can be whole wheat, white, rye, or combination)
1/2 cup brown sugar
2 tsp. baking soda
1 tsp. baking powder
2 tsp. cinnamon
1/2 cup wheat germ
1/2 cup ground flax seeds
2 cups grated carrots or zucchini
1/2 cup raisins
1/2 cup chopped nuts or seeds
1/2 cup coconut or 1 tsp. coconut extract
1 apple grated
2 eggs
1 cup soy milk
1/4 cup olive oil
2 tsp. vanilla extract
1/2 cup no-fat yogurt

In a large mixing bowl combine the dry ingredients. In a smaller bowl, beat the eggs, oil, vanilla, and yogurt together, and stir in the carrots, raisins, nuts, coconut, and apple. Combine the wet ingredients with the dry ingredients and stir until well mixed. Spoon into lightly-buttered muffin tins. Bake for 40 minutes at 350 degrees.

Will make twelve large nutritious delicious muffins. Enjoy!

David had deliberately planned his next visit at the same time as Mary Ann's yoga class. He was in luck, and grinned broadly as he saw her at the juice bar.

"Are you finished already or are you just starting your workout?" he asked."

I've had a swim already, but I'm planning on attending a Body Blast class. Care to join me?" she replied.

"And Body Blast is what, exactly?" asked David.

"Oh, it's a one-hour class that Karley teaches, which combines strength training and conditioning, including wind sprints, push-ups, sit-ups, and core strengthening." David decided to join the mostly female, spandex-clad group but made the wise decision to stick to the Level One variations on the exercises. He was humbled by how difficult it was to keep in step with the fit and strong women, and recognized it would be some time before he caught up to them.

After the class, David and Mary Ann decided to go for a walk at Spanish Banks near UBC. "Since we last talked, I've been thinking about the role of spirituality in healing," began David hesitantly. "I've been trying to slow down my mind, pay attention to the moment, enjoy the great outdoors, and think positively about the future. What are your own strategies?"

Mary Ann thought for a moment. "I don't want to drift aimlessly like a twig in a stream, and sometimes I'm not exactly sure where I'm headed, or what God's plan for me is. So I start each morning with a simple prayer:

> *Lord as I begin another day, help me to live as you desire. Keep me ever aware of your presence and ever alert to opportunities to serve you and the people I meet. I wish to make the best use of this day. Guide my steps that I may not go astray. Amen.*

They walked in silence for a while. David took some deep breaths of the saltwater breeze coming off the ocean. The sun was going down and the clouds were various shades of pink and purple and orange. He said, "Wow, what an awesome evening."

"We use that word a lot," Mary Ann said, "so that it sometimes loses its meaning. But you are right; walking along this beach, often fills me with a sense of wonder and awe. I heard the Archbishop use those words recently. We are not Roman Catholic, but Erika's friend Sophia is. Last weekend, she celebrated her confirmation, and we attended the Mass. The Archbishop told them of the seven gifts of the Holy Spirit. I thought it would be wonderful if each of us were blessed with these gifts."

"I'll try to remember them. There is the gift of *wisdom* to make good choices. The gift of *courage* to live our faith and remain true to our convictions even when challenged. The gift of *knowledge*, and the continual desire to seek knowledge. The gift of *understanding*. The gift of *right judgment*: while we are urged not to judge others, it is important to be discerning. The gift of *reverence*, and finally (and this is my favourite) the gift of *wonder and awe* at this remarkable creation."

"Those are amazing gifts," David had to admit. "And you are correct that they are worth striving for. That actually reminds me of a Bible reading from my wedding. For some reason it stuck with me. It was about being ambitious for the higher gifts and went on to say that love is always patient and kind and that we are nothing without love.[61] I'm not a church guy, as you know, but I remember thinking that I really wanted to experience that kind of pure and fulfilling love—and strive for excellence in life—and in my marriage. The gifts you mentioned would help me reach those goals. I think I can use some help from up above, as I don't seem to have done that well on my own—but I have to admit I probably did not hold up my end of the deal. I can't say that I put my partner first. A marriage does not work if only one partner is committed to it." David mused aloud.

I'm really not sure what the future holds for me, but I've been re-examining my direction after my heart attack. I feel a spiritual awakening, and perhaps that begins with experiencing the wonder and awe of nature in all its glory, such as this sunset."

Mary Ann agreed that a silent walk outdoors was when she felt closest to God and was often the time when the best ideas would pop into her head. "I hope you have the courage to explore your own faith, David, and that you will take the opportunity to make that journey," said

---

[61] 1Cor 13:4—13

Mary Ann. "Personally, I like the traditions of the Christian church I attend and find it a comfortable home for my faith as it allows me to deepen my relationship with Jesus. But I also admire spiritual leaders like the Buddha, and Gandhi. And I was lucky enough to hear the Dalai Lama speak in Vancouver. As best as I can sum up, he said that many people may not believe in religion or rebirth, but everyone appreciates honesty, compassion, and loving kindness. The big difference that I see among the World Religions, however, is that only Jesus claimed to be God. That makes him either a liar, a madman, or someone that I want to know to be close to God."

Mary Ann looked at her watch and laughed. "I'd best be getting back," she said. "Erika and her sitter will be wondering where I've got to. I've enjoyed our walk together," she smiled.

*Prayer is not asking. It is a longing of the soul. It is a daily admission of one's weakness. It is better in prayer to have a heart without words than words without a heart.*

**Mohandas Karamchand Gandhi** (1869–1948). Political and spiritual leader of India. Founder of the Indian Independence Movement through non-violent civil disobedience.[62]

A week later, David was getting ready to leave the Peninsula Club after a class when he saw a familiar face at the other end of a

[62] Gandhi is often referred to as *Mahatma* not because that's his first name, but because it is a title that bestows honour. It is derived from the Sanskrit words *maha* meaning "great" and *atma* meaning "soul."

mop cleaning the locker room. "Hey, Raj! How have you been?" he said to his former roommate from the cardiology ward.

"I'm good, David," replied Raj with a smile. "You remember I was working at St. Luke's for twelve years until the restructuring and then became a guest on the cardiac ward when I had my valve job done. Dr. Schreiber had me doing a cardiac rehab program for three months after the surgery, and when I started this job, I scored a membership to the club, which allows me to continue the work outs. I'm finished in a few minutes; I can meet you at 'Get Juiced' if you have time."

David went up to the lounge and ordered a couple of smoothies—a Matcha Monsoon for Raj and the CBC (Cabbage Beets Celery) for himself.

The two men compared notes on the dietary and lifestyle changes they had been making since their hospitalizations. Raj mentioned that he had attended a yoga class led by a young woman who could have been a drill sergeant in a previous life. She lined the students up in straight lines on their mats and ran the class with precision, tolerating no margin of error in the execution of the various poses. Raj found it curious, however, that she would often slag the medical profession during her class. As far as she was concerned, no doctor would ever recommend yoga for their patients, as they got paid by the number of pills they prescribed! He had wanted to tell her that he strongly disagreed with her perspective, but decided to just let the misguided comments go and concentrate on his pose and his breathing. He'd look for another instructor the next time.

Raj looked well; he had lost some weight, but more importantly had lost his midline girth. Dr. Schreiber told him that his waist had to be smaller than his hips, but unfortunately, at that time, his belly had hung well over his belt. "The doc was funny. He told me it was the worst kind of hangover!" laughed Raj.

"It was not complicated to reach my goal—but it sure was not easy. My wife and I visited a nutritionist (as my dietician preferred to be called) and together we modified my favourite traditional recipes and also added some new ones. We tried to eliminate all sugar and flour products, but found that this was an unrealistic goal."

"I also worked with an Ayurvedic physician to find my dosha (or constitutional body type) and found that I could develop a palatable diet that reduced my weight. I began to see the light when I recognized that it was not only the type of food but the quantity that had to be modified. "While it is critically important to be selective about the food we put into our mouths, it is caloric restriction that results in weight loss," he said, accurately quoting his doctor.

"And guess what, David," continued Raj. "I felt too tired from my job to exercise much before. Now I'm working with a trainer at the club and am committed to getting sixty minutes of fairly vigorous exercise at least five times a week. As my job is quite physical—which counts too—I'm getting plenty of exercise nearly every day."

"I used to worry a lot and got stressed out over things I could not change," confided Raj. "A friend who attended AA (Alcoholics Anonymous) meetings gave me a copy of the Serenity Prayer that has taught me to concentrate my efforts on what I can change," he continued. "Now I try to decide which battles to fight and which ones to walk away from. When I feel myself digging in I think—*is this a hill I'm prepared to die on*—and then I can let it go."

In the past, when he had tried to lose a few pounds, Raj admitted that he had become so hungry that he ate more than he would have if he were not on the latest diet. After his wake-up call on the cardiac ward, he had a sense of urgency. It was not easy eating less. He experienced headaches, nausea, tremulousness, sweats, and a sense of impending doom for the first week as he withdrew from many of his bad food habits. Gradually, he felt more alert and energetic, and he noticed that even his hearing and vision seemed sharper.

"I had never bothered to read labels and found all the recommendations regarding healthy foods to be confusing," admitted Raj. "However, the cardiologist had a good way of putting it all in perspective. 'Only eat things from the ground and the ocean' were his parting words. That made it simple. You can't go wrong with veggies, grain, and fish."

Raj was on his way to a piano lesson, but promised to e-mail David to stay in touch. David checked his e-mails that evening.

> Great to see you again, David. I was pleased to hear about some of the changes you have been making. I'm also sending you the Serenity Prayer we talked about. Be well, Raj.

**Serenity Prayer**
God grant me the serenity
to accept the things I cannot change;
courage to change the things I can;
and wisdom to know the difference.

........................................................................

Remembering his conversation with Mary Ann about the role of spirituality, David asked Dr. Osler at his next appointment if he were aware of any cases of healing that were inexplicable. "There are certainly well-documented cases of spontaneous remissions as well as of miracle cures, but I'm not sure what they can be attributed to," replied the physician.

"One tragic case I was personally involved in has elements that I can't explain. There was a twelve-year-old boy in our community who was good at everything he tried; he was very bright and although popular at school, was genuinely modest and even shy. And he was passionate about bicycling. Let's call him 'Drew.'"

"One day Drew was cycling back from school with a friend when he lost his balance on uneven pavement and struck the back of his head on the curb. Although Drew always wore a helmet, for some reason he did not have it on that afternoon. He had a brief loss of consciousness, vomited, and then made his way home with his buddy at his side. His mother took one look at him and immediately called an ambulance. At our local hospital, a CT scan showed he had a skull fracture and was bleeding into his brain. Drew was transferred to BC Children's Hospital in Vancouver, where, despite heroic efforts in the ER, he died of his injuries."

"As Chair of the Quality Assurance Committee of our local hospital, it was my responsibility to review the case. I also got in touch with the family to express my condolences on behalf of the hospital. As a result of the conversation, Drew's dad became my patient. He was, of course, devastated by the loss of his son; he knew this was a scar on his soul that would never heal."

"Perhaps because of the medication we had initiated at his first appointment, the talk we had, and through the tincture of time, the dad was feeling somewhat better by the next time I saw him. He had an unusual request. He wanted to know if I could find out exactly when the resuscitation of his son had started. At one point during the ordeal, Drew's dad had been overcome by an unusual feeling and had noticed the sky brightening. Although it was sunny, the sky appeared to be opening briefly as it would on a cloudy day. He had glanced at his watch. Later, Drew's dad had found out that Drew's brother had been in Drew's room when the door slammed at that exact moment, even though it was not windy and no one else was nearby.

My patient recounted a recent dream in which he saw Drew and asked him about heaven. "It's beautiful, Dad," was the reply. The experience was so vivid that he couldn't be sure whether it was a dream or whether he had actually seen his son again.

We talked about how the dream had brought him some comfort and that the intensity of his grief was a sign of the depth of the bond he shared with Drew. "From my standpoint," concluded Osler, "it was another example of how things that we experience can't all be explained through the laws of physics and time. 'The non-local mind' seems to have a role to play in healing."[63]

---

[63] For a discussion of the non-local mind, see: Dossey, Larry, 1999, *Reinventing Medicine—Beyond Mind-Body to a New Era of Healing*, Harper San Francisco

# CHAPTER 8

*People rarely succeed unless they have fun in what they are doing.*

**Andrew Carnegie** (1835–1919)

Scottish-born industrialist and philanthropist who immigrated as a child to the United States and earned his fortune as a steel baron.

Mary Ann and David arranged to meet at the Peninsula Club for a yoga class. Afterwards, they had an invigorating "Green Supreme" energy drink and went for a walk on the river bank. At one point, Mary Ann mentioned that she had wanted to become a surgeon but because of life circumstances became a nurse. "I don't feel I am reaching my full potential," she mused. "I could make a greater difference in the world if I were a surgeon. I'd like to help cancer patients, get involved with teaching medical students and residents, as well as volunteer my skills in the Third World."

David suggested to her that these were noble goals but that she need not be at all disappointed if she did not achieve them. "Bloom where you are planted," he said. "Play the cards that you have been dealt, not the cards you wish you had. It is important to set your standards high and work hard to achieve your goals; too often people do not reach their potential in life because they are not willing to put in the effort. However, it is also essential to put your heart and soul into what you are doing."

"Let me tell you about a trip we had to Germany a while back," continued David. "When I was eighteen, our whole family went on a trip to Germany because my mom and dad sang in a choir and they had booked a concert tour. We travelled from town to town on a tour bus. The bus driver, who made a point of being called our 'coach driver'—to differentiate himself from a city bus driver—was an energetic young man named Sascha. He explained that city bus drivers work regular shifts, do not communicate with their passengers and sleep in their own beds every night. He, on the other hand, in the previous year had stayed in hotels 240 nights, driven through the night 60 times and only slept in his own bed 65 nights. He was a highly-skilled driver who was able to get a big tour bus down narrow streets and was full of interesting information about the sights we were taking in. What he did not know he looked up, and he treated every question he received with respect."

"Sascha was an important part of what made that trip enjoyable. Normally, a bus driver is not on the highest rung of the ladder of life, as Dick van Dyke once sang about chimney sweeps in Mary Poppins. Yet here was a bright and articulate man who chose to bring his all to what he was doing, and by doing so enriched the lives of those around him and made a positive difference in the world. As it turned out, Sascha's father owned the tour bus business and started his son off on the same road. At the age of twenty-six, Sascha already owned two buses and was on his way to a lucrative career by doing what he enjoyed and did well."

Mary Ann smiled. "That's a great story, David. It is so important to put vigour and passion in your work. I do love what I do, but at times I think I could have done a lot more. Maybe I still will."

"I feel that you are making a tremendous difference in the world by caring for sick and injured patients at St. Luke's," replied David. "Your genuine concern and excellent care touched me and comforted me during my hospitalization. I attribute my recovery as much to the care of the nurses as to the skillful interventions of my cardiologist, Dr. Schreiber."

"Have you thought of teaching and mentoring other nurses in order to broaden your career and disseminate your wisdom?" asked David. "You could continue to work in the ICU as well to expand your field of expertise."

Mary Ann looked genuinely pleased at the interest David was showing in her work. "Thank you, David. I will take your advice to heart."

As they parted, David realized how much he was enjoying Mary Ann's company; he had found himself thinking about her when he was riding his bike or relaxing at home, and looked for opportunities and situations when he could cross paths with her again. That evening, he turned once again to his book; reading it before bed was becoming a nightly ritual.

*If you are called to be a street sweeper, sweep streets even as Michelangelo painted, or Beethoven composed music, or Shakespeare wrote poetry. Sweep streets so well that all the hosts of heaven and earth will pause to say, 'Here lived a great street sweeper who did his job well.'*

**Martin Luther King, Jr.**

**HABIT SEVEN: ENJOYMENT OF WORK**

When we follow our passions, life takes on new meaning. When we are involved in a pursuit that really matters to us and resonates with our personal values, we feel a sense of satisfaction in a profound way. We become absorbed in this activity and time seems to stand still. Fortunate indeed is the person who is able to develop their passion into their work. Almost any passion can become one's livelihood and in many cases can be profitable as well as enjoyable.

> It is important to allow yourself to follow your passions even if this is not your employment. Your job may provide your livelihood, but your hobbies and passions provide your life. You cannot let the things you want to do always take a back seat to the things you have to do. At the same time, it is important to bring a sense of pride and passion to whatever your job may be.

David knew he should be getting back to work sometime soon, but in reality he was starting to enjoy not working and sometimes he played with the idea that he would never return to the office. Throughout law school, articles, and then as a young associate who worked hard to impress the partners, David's own thoughts and ideas had simply passed him by or been placed on the back burner. He was too busy to contemplate what mattered most because he was too occupied with getting ahead. Now, for the first time since he was a kid lying on his back and gazing at cloud formations, he felt free to daydream or think of nothing in particular.

He was starting to feel guilty about having kept *12 Habits* for such a long time, so he took out the business card he had found in it and phoned the number. He was somewhat surprised that his mid-afternoon call was answered after a few rings. "Sanjay here," was the greeting in a warm voice that sounded vaguely familiar.

"Hello, Sanjay. My name is David McKenzie, and I found your book in a taxi a few months ago when I was coming home from St. Luke's Hospital." said David by way of introduction. "I'm sorry I didn't call earlier to arrange to return it to you."

"It's kind of you to ring me up," said Sanjay. "Please keep it. Did you enjoy reading it?" he asked.

"I haven't quite finished it yet," replied David. "I am finding it truly transformational. What is the Magna Vita Institute, by the way?"

"It's an organization devoted to living one's life to the fullest," replied Sanjay. "If you feel like getting together with me sometime, we can talk about it further."

David thanked Sanjay for his offer. "I'd be very interested. I'll get back to you after I've finished the book."

*I try to treat everyone I meet as an old friend. This gives me a genuine feeling of happiness.*

**The Dalai Lama.** His Holiness the 14th Dalai Lama, Tenzin Gyatso, was born in 1935. Recognized at the age of two as the reincarnation of the 13th Dalai Lama, he is both head of state and spiritual leader of Tibet.

**How to be Happy**

Nearly everyone desires to be happy. The pursuit of happiness has been the subject of books and movies too numerous to name. How to define happiness and how to achieve it, however, remain elusive goals. According to Aristotle, "Happiness is the whole aim and end of human existence."

He described four levels of happiness: instant gratification, gratification through achievement, gratification through contribution to others, and transcendent gratification. In this highest level of happiness, we live more consistently from a place of purpose and truth, using our signature strengths to serve others, and working - in various and creative ways- for the good of the world.

*That makes happiness seem altruistic and rather elusive,* thought David. *Whatever happened to just having fun?* But he read on.

> "Consider that some things that make us happy are out of our control. Growing up in a caring family, having enough to eat, having the opportunity to go school and study a desired profession, and being generally healthy are all important to our happiness but are often taken for granted. These factors of happiness may be better described as "luck."
>
> Other "wins" may also make us happy but are not in our control. For example, having our name drawn in a lottery, not getting a parking ticket when the meter expired, or getting invited out on a date or to a dinner party will make us feel happy even though we had no hand in making it happen.
>
> There are attributes of happy people, however, that can be learned and practiced and contribute more consistently to happiness rather than hoping for good luck. Much of this has to do with our attitude. It is important to *care* about others and genuinely make the effort do something in which the beneficiary is another person. This demonstrates a belief in something bigger than ourselves. Doing things for others, and always doing our best, gives purpose and meaning to life, which leads to a sense of fulfillment. This feeling that we are doing what we are meant to be doing results in a deep level of

satisfaction and happiness. Another attitude that can be practised is that of optimism and sufficiency. When we see the glass as half full and feel truly grateful for all that we have, it allows us to move ahead with confidence and happiness and leaves little room for regret.

> Dan Baker, PhD, is a Family Business and Organizational Consultant. He is an Executive Coach and was the Founder of the Life Enhancement Centre at Canyon Ranch, a health spa outside Tucson, AZ, where he worked from 1986 to 1997. The author met him there while attending a workshop on "Examining Integrative Medicine with Dr. Andrew Weil" in 1997. In *What Happy People Know*, Dan Baker discusses 12 Points to Happiness: 1. Love, 2. Optimism, 3. Courage, 4. Sense of Freedom, 5. Proactive, 6. Security, 7. Health, 8. Spirituality, 9. Altruism, 10. Perspective, 11. Humour, 12. Purpose.

The human soul fundamentally yearns to be "happy." Moreover, it is apparent that the definitions of *happiness* and *health* are essentially the same—and the attributes of happy and healthy people are very similar. Both imply wholeness and balance. To have the best chances of being healthy and happy, it is critical that we pay attention to diet and exercise, and just as importantly, to social and spiritual connections, in order to live lives of purpose, meaning, value, and ultimate satisfaction.

Marriage also seems to be a key to happiness. While there are numerous conflicting studies on the role of marital status on happiness, and while not all married people are happy, one researcher has found that married people are happier than those who were never married and those who are divorced. His study reveals that marriage is a more potent happiness indicator than job satisfaction, finances, and community.[64]

**One minute message**

If you can't always do what you love, then learn to love what you do.

Ensure that you do at least *one thing* each day that you are passionate about, that gives you *joy,* and that resonates with who you are. Be grateful for what you have—foster an *attitude of gratitude.*

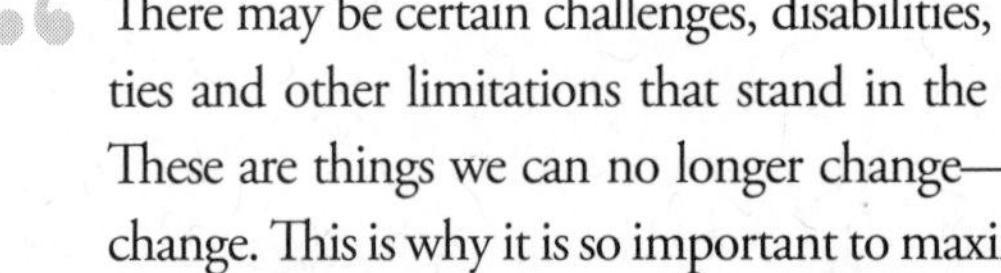

"There may be certain challenges, disabilities, lost opportunities and other limitations that stand in the way of success. These are things we can no longer change—or could never change. This is why it is so important to maximize the potential we have. Our goal—in fact, our obligation—is to live our lives to their fullest potential, to be the best we are capable of becoming. When we start to think about reaching our full potential and the purpose of our life we begin to focus on what is truly important. At that point, more superficial goals and desires tend to evaporate, and we become "real."

---

[64] Seligman, Martin—Psychologist and Author of Authentic Happiness: Using the New Positive Psychology to Realize Your Potential for Lasting Fulfillment (2002) and Learned Optimism, How to Change Your Mind and Your Life (2004)—is dedicated to making the world a happier place.

# CHAPTER 9

*A good laugh and a long sleep are the best cures in the doctor's book.*

**Irish Proverb**

Although Jessica was outwardly cool in his presence, David yearned to spend time with her and their two kids. During his recuperation, he had taken the time to ponder his priorities. He knew now that he could not live without his family, and that he had been far too cavalier in his relationship with his wife. He realized how precious Jessica was to him and vowed to no longer take her for granted if he could be given the opportunity to prove his love. He left a message on her phone to invite her and Adam and Rebecca to his place for a salmon barbeque.

He was a little surprised that Jessica called him back about an hour later to accept the invitation. "It's a novel concept, you cooking the dinner," she said lightly. "I'm looking forward to it."

David took the opportunity to tell her about his new fitness regime. "That's good to hear, David," she said quietly. "I'm only sorry it took a health crisis to get you to the gym and on your bike."

"And you?" asked David. "Are you keeping well?"

Jessica explained that she had just been working out with a friend. Cathie was a phys ed teacher whom she had met while covering a maternity leave. Cathie's husband had been a professional athlete and now owned a chain of fitness stores. The couple had built a well-equipped gym in their home. "I can't believe what a difference it's made in my life," enthused Jessica. "Cathie's got me into power walks and circuit weight training—the kind of stuff I never thought I wanted to do. I'm in better shape now than I was in college days."

There had been an exceptionally good run of sockeye salmon that season and David had been given the opportunity to go fishing with his urologist friend, Herman. As a result, he had a few choice sides of salmon in his freezer, and decided he would impress Jessica and the kids with a tasty and healthy meal. He made a salad with mixed organic greens to which he added avocado slices, papaya, caramelized pecans, and fresh blueberries and strawberries that were still in season. He dressed it with his own maple balsamic vinaigrette dressing. He found a recipe for Arborio rice with broccoli rosettes, dried cranberries, and sweet white onions to go with the salmon.

He went all out and cleaned up the apartment and even picked up some flowers and candles to create a warm and cozy atmosphere. The most time-consuming preparation was the cleaning of the barbeque, which the previous tenant had not paid much attention to.

Once the family had arrived, he lightly drizzled the salmon fillets with a citrus mustard glaze, and placed them on the grill. David was careful to not overcook the fish. He and Jessica washed down this feast with a glass of pinot noir from his favourite Okanagan winery, along with some lightly carbonated water. For dessert, he had made a wholesome peach cobbler with organic oats that he served with low-fat yogurt. As Adam and Rebecca dug into second helpings, Jessica turned to David. "I can't believe you're the same man I married!" she laughed. When it was time to take the kids home, she gave him a warm hug.

"Could I come home to tuck the kids in and read them a bedtime story?" asked David. Jessica declined, saying, "Let's not spoil this wonderful evening, and besides, the kids have been reading on their own for years." Then she gave him a peck on the cheek. "Thanks again for dinner. We'll get out of your hair now and let you tidy up your kitchen."

David put on some music. He was feeling more than a bit sorry for himself that he had fussed all day to make a great meal, and now he was left to clean everything up as well. Meanwhile, Jessica had been wined and dined, wiped her mouth and left! That was so unfair—but then he realized with chagrin that he had behaved in a similar manner for years in their marriage. With that insight he reflected on what a fabulous time they had had as a family, and how this evening had been worth the effort he had put into making it happen.

The next day David had a follow-up appointment with his doctor. He spoke to Osler about his progress in the cardiac rehab program. He was stable on his meds, eating well, and exercising for at least one hour, at least four times a week.

"Is there something else I should be doing to reduce my risk of having another heart attack?" asked David.

Osler smiled. "You're one of my most motivated patients, David. It's very important that you keep up your lifestyle changes and that you remain on appropriate doses of medications, because high-tech procedures like angioplasty may not benefit patients who have stable coronary artery disease if they are already on optimal medical therapy."[65]

"Of course, in your case, you required an angioplasty procedure as a blockage was discovered when you arrived at St. Luke's after your heart attack. Now you need to focus on maintaining your lifestyle changes, hitting your lipid and blood pressure targets with medications as required, and trying to fit that into a

---

[65] Boden, William et al, for the COURAGE Trial Research Group, 2007, Optimal Medical Therapy with or without PCI for Stable Coronary Disease, *New England Journal of Medicine,* Volume 356: 1503–1516, April 12

normal work and social life. You also need to find things that you are passionate about and that make you leap out of bed in the morning."

"What do you like most about your own work?" asked David.

Osler told him that he enjoyed the challenge of helping individuals with serious medical conditions who were motivated to improve their outcomes. "But I'm still involved with our maternity clinic and take call for the group once a week," he told David. "It's such a privilege to share the intimate moment of childbirth with a family. I feel blessed to be able to make a living doing what I love to do. As I get older, though," he had to admit, "I do find it harder to go without sleep and try to function in the office the next day. I appreciate more than ever that sleep rocks!"

"I hear you", agreed David. "I used to get headaches and felt grumpy and sluggish after I pulled an all-nighter in college or stayed up way too late preparing a case. Since I made it a priority to get sufficient sleep, I feel more energetic, mentally sharper, and notice that I get fewer colds as well. I recently read that the nuclear accident at Chernobyl, the near-meltdown at Three Mile Island, the environmentally disastrous oil spill by the Exxon Valdez, and the loss of the space shuttle Challenger were all caused by people who had too little sleep. It turns out that Edison's invention of the light bulb made us more productive but robbed each of us of more than 500 hours of sleep a year!"[66]

*To sleep, perchance to dream, aye—there's the rub.*

**William Shakespeare** (1564–1616) Hamlet, Act 3, scene 1

---

[66] Coren, Stanley, 1996, *Sleep Thieves, An Eye-opening Exploration into the Science and Mysteries of Sleep*. New York: The Free Press. A book that deals with some of the fascinating facts associated with sleep, as well as the serious implications of a society that is running on too little sleep.

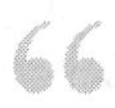

## HABIT EIGHT: SLEEP WELL

Natural sleep cycles are controlled by your *circadian rhythm*. This is an internal biological clock that regulates a variety of biochemical, physiological, and behavioural processes according to an approximate twenty-four-hour period. These affect body temperature, alertness, appetite, hormone levels as well as sleep timing. Circadian rhythm sleep disorders occur when one's internal biological clock does not set one's sleep-wake cycles with the usual times required for work, school, and social activities. This results in sleepiness and wakefulness occurring at times that do not match the required times of alertness. This can be due to external factors such as jet lag and shift work, or can be symptomatic of stress or depression, or due to an intrinsic sleep disorder.

Certain health conditions have been found to occur more frequently at specific times of day, demonstrating their relationship to circadian rhythm. Lack of sleep can trigger epileptic seizures. Strokes and heart attacks occur more often in the last third of the night.

People with sleep apnea, or interrupted breathing during sleep, are eight times more likely to have a motor vehicle accident and three to four times more likely to suffer a heart attack. If you stay awake just seventeen hours your brain behaves as though you have a blood alcohol level of 0.05, the legal limit for drinking and driving in most European countries and the level the Canadian Medical Associations defines as the level of impairment. (In September 2010, the legal blood alcohol limit in British Columbia was reduced from 0.08 to 0.05 to reduce the carnage from alcohol related motor vehicle accidents.)

A single all-nighter or a week of four or five hours of sleep per night impairs your mental and physical performance as if you had a blood alcohol level of about 0.1. Language, memory, and planning skills drop. Athletic performance drops. Specifically, you may experience reduced motor function, cardiovascular performance, endurance, coordination, and delayed visual and auditory reaction times.

**Stages of alcohol intoxication based on Blood Alcohol Content** (g/100 ml of blood) 0.01–0.03—nearly Normal, 0.03–0.12—impaired: euphoric with reduced judgment and concentration, 0.08—legally drunk in most parts of Canada and the USA, 0.09–0.25—impaired balance, perception, and comprehension, 0.25–0.40—vomiting, incontinence, loss of most motor function, reduced pain sensation and level of consciousness, 0.40–0.50—unconsciousness, respiratory arrest and possible death. (Radford University, Virginia, 1996)

Even a few weeks of insufficient sleep increases blood pressure and stress hormones, worsens glucose control and increases appetite. Lack of sleep releases less of the pleasure hormone serotonin in your brain. To compensate, you try to increase those levels with foods like sugar or with harmful substances like tobacco or stimulants such as coffee. This is why chronic sleep deprivation can result in weight gain.[67]

[67] Fleming, Jonathan, 2007, Professor of Psychiatry and Co-Director of the Sleep Disorders Program at the University of British Columbia Hospital, Quoted in: *Lack of Sleep Linked to Numerous Problems—Even Disasters: Highly Complex*, The National Post, 15 March, page A16, article by Jenny Lee

Insomnia is associated with fatigue, malaise, lack of concentration and motivation, impaired memory and social functioning, difficulty in school or at work, mood disturbance, daytime sleepiness, high blood pressure, tension headaches, poor judgment making one prone to accidents or errors at work or while driving, and a reduced immune response resulting in infections and illness.

Interestingly, these symptoms of insomnia are also symptoms of stress. This indicates the reciprocal relationship between sleep deprivation and stress-related symptoms. In the same way, increasing the amount we sleep can reduce symptoms of stress.

If these were not enough reasons to get a good night's rest, sleep may also be an important part of cancer prevention. Poor sleep appears to disrupt patterns of the hormones cortisol and melatonin. Cortisol is a stress hormone that is triggered during anxiety or stress and reduced with rest and sleep. It may play a role in cancer development. Melatonin is produced by the pineal gland, a light-sensitive gland at the base of the brain. In order to optimize melatonin production, it is advisable to dim lights in the house by 9:00 PM and to be in bed by 10:00 PM.

Melatonin may have antioxidant properties that help to prevent cancer-causing damage to the cells of the body. These hormonal disruptions could reduce a person's defences against the development or worsening of cancer.[68] The cumulative effects of inadequate sleep

---

[68] Sephton S., Spiegel D., 2003, Circadian disruption in cancer: a neuroendocrine-immune pathway from stress to disease? Brain Behavior and Immunity. Oct; 17(5):321–8.

reduce life expectancy to a similar degree as smoking a pack of cigarettes a day.

Good quality sleep significantly helps boost the immune system to the extent that that adequate sleep promotes optimal healing. Stress hormones are metabolized during sleep, which is why people who sleep well have reduced anxiety and depression. Sleep improves memory and facilitates learning, which is why we feel sharper and more alert in the morning—or after a nap—making these optimal times to study.

Humans generally like to sleep seven to nine hours but the range is from five to eleven hours a night. In contrast, cats sleep twelve hours a day. Giraffes need less than two.

It takes more than one good night's sleep to fully recover from a few days of sleep deficit. Work with your circadian rhythm and go to bed earlier rather than sleeping in, and if you need to take a nap, try to do so in the late morning or early afternoon rather than later in the day.

The optimal period of sleep, according to several studies, is seven to eight hours. Less sleep can double one's risk of death due to cardiovascular disease, and is a risk factor for weight gain, hypertension, and Type 2 Diabetes. Sleeping fewer than six hours a night has been shown to reduce blood flow to the brain. Tanking up on sleep if we have not been getting enough is tremendously energizing. However, consistently oversleeping is related to reduced productivity and an increased mortality rate compared to those who regularly got seven or eight hours of refreshing sleep. [69]

It is not exactly clear why, but if one gets less sleep than

---

[69] McLean's Magazine reported this research on October 8, 2007

required, or if sleep quality is poor, it increases arterial aging and the risk of heart attacks. It is also important that the sleep we get is continuous; although one can feel refreshed after a quick nap, it takes about two-and-a-half hours of straight sleep before it becomes truly restorative. As humans age, we tend to sleep less. Newborn babies often sleep up to twenty hours a day in the first days of life. As they grow, their sleep requirement gradually drops to ten to twelve hours, and then around adolescence it drops to eight to ten hours (although, given the chance, a lot of teens could sleep in for at least twelve hours). Most adults make do with six to eight hours. As adults get older, they tend to have a harder time sleeping. This is due to several factors, including that most retired people are not as physically active as they were when they worked. Furthermore, seniors may have chronic pain, heart disease, depression and other health conditions ("comorbidities") that rob them of sleep. A national sleep survey conducted in the United States concluded that the sleep complaints common in older adults are often secondary to their underlying comorbidities, rather than to aging per se.[70]

**Assessment for Adequate Sleep**

1. Do you need an alarm clock to wake up? Most of us set alarm clocks in order to awake on time. Frequently, we are still tired when the alarm clock goes off. This usually indicates that we have not had enough sleep.

[70] Foley, D, et.al., 2004, Sleep disturbances and chronic disease in older adults: Results of the 2003 National Sleep Foundation Sleep in America Survey. *Journal of Psychosomatic Research*, May;56(5):497-502.

2. Do you feel well rested in the morning? After a good night's sleep, we should be ready to bounce out of bed and face the day with vigour and energy.
3. How is your daytime energy? Is caffeine required to start the day? Do you feel tired in the afternoon, requiring coffee or a nap?
4. How much sleep do you get on weekends or when you don't need to get up early? Sleeping in for a few hours is a sign we have been sleep deprived during other days.
5. How quickly do you fall asleep? Sleep latency is normally fifteen to twenty minutes. If we fall asleep upon hitting the pillow this is usually a sign that we are sleep deprived. Longer latency indicates insomnia—usually because the mind wanders and does not allow sleep to occur.
6. An objective way to assess your sleep quality is by completing the Epworth Sleepiness Scale, which is available on line.[71]

**One minute message**

Sleep is an active process that recharges our bodies and enhances our minds. *Sleep deprivation* leads to a *decrease* in learning, memory, energy, performance, and healing, as well as an *increase* in accidents, obesity, hypertension and depression. For sleep to be restorative it must be sufficiently deep, long, and regular. Aim for a peaceful eight hours every night.

[71] Dr. Murray Johns, developed the Epworth Sleepiness Scale at Epworth Hospital, Melbourne, Australia in 1990. It is an often used, validated score which is available on Dr. Johns's official website: epworthsleepinessscale.com.

If you are not getting good sleep, see your doctor to rule out a medical condition and then adopt a consistent evening ritual to get into the habit of sleeping well.

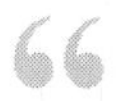

Although most of us function well with less, several studies have shown that our natural sleep cycle is probably eight to ten hours of sleep per night. Primitive tribes without electricity generally sleep this length of time. Researchers working in the high Arctic in constant darkness have no time cues. In these circumstances, by checking when they log onto and off of computers when they awake and before they fall asleep it has been determined that eight to ten hours of sleep is the usual pattern for them.

Young adults who get good sleep should not need naps during the daytime. If a power nap is required, it should be taken in the early afternoon, typically for ten or fifteen minutes and for no more than half an hour so as not to interfere with sleep at night.

Light also has an important role in sleep. Bright light in the morning promotes good sleep at night. This is in part because of the light stimulating the pineal gland behind the eyes, which releases melatonin. High lux lights used in the daytime improve moods and alertness and have been used to treat Seasonal Affective Disorder (winter blues). Light therapy can also be used by shift workers to delay sleep or to treat jet lag. Bright light in the evening delays sleep.

While medications can be used to promote sleep, long term use is habit forming and should be avoided. A study out of Boston, Massachusetts showed that Cognitive

Behavioural Therapy (CBT) was more effective than pharmacotherapy in the treatment of chronic insomnia in young and middle-aged adults. They concluded that this was a safe and effective therapy that should be used more often in the treatment of chronic insomnia.[72]

Consider using a journal to document how much you sleep, especially if you have a busy travel schedule. During the 2010 NBA playoffs, legendary basketball great—two-time NBA MVP and the player with the highest shooting percentage—Steve Nash was interviewed about his training. Nash indicated that he kept a Sleep Diary to ensure that he got adequate rest, and also refrained from eating sugary foods and other refined carbohydrates.[73] There are many people taller or even more athletic than Steve Nash who do not excel at basketball as he does. Motivation, determination, and the discipline to stick to an effective training regime yield consistent results and make the difference between mediocrity and excellence. In the same way, each of us needs to modify the variables in our lives that we can control to optimize our potential and make the best of what we have.

## Sleep Hygiene: Tips for Getting Better Sleep

1. Establish a consistent bedtime routine, and try to go to bed around the same time every night. Even more

---

[72] Jacobs, G.D., et. al., 2004, Cognitive Behavior Therapy and Pharmacotherapy for Insomnia: A Randomized Controlled Trial and Direct Comparison, *Archives of Internal Medicine*, Vol.164 No. 17:1888–1896.

[73] Cluff, Rick, host of The Early Edition on CBC Radio One, Vancouver, read this story on May 17, 2010.

importantly, *anchor your rising time* so that you get up approximately the same time each day—even on weekends. This is more predictable than when you go to bed and will not affect your circadian rhythm to the extent that sleeping in does.

2. The room should be cool and dark. Your bed should be comfortable; invest in a good mattress and pillow. Fix the squeaky bed frame that keeps you awake and drives you crazy.
3. Take the time to relax in the evening before going to bed. Dim the lights by nine or ten PM. A warm bath can be part of your bedtime ritual. Avoid watching TV an hour before going to sleep—especially the evening news, as the intense stimulation and negative images can delay the onset of restful sleep.
4. Set aside fifteen minutes or so before you go to bed as your "worry time" or problem solving time. Take a note pad and write out all the things that you are concerned about as well as possible solutions. When you have exhausted this list, allow yourself to be "off duty" for the night and put these matters to rest. You can leave the notepad by your bedside, and if you cannot get a specific concern out of your mind, then write it on the notepad and deal with it in the morning.
5. Create the habit of going to bed with the intent to sleep. If you are not drowsy, do not go to bed yet. If you are tossing and turning and unable to sleep, get up and go to another room. Do something mentally stimulating such as reading, or writing a letter, solving a cross word puzzle or Sudoku, rather than

watching television. When you feel tired, go back to bed with the expectation that you will have a good sleep. It's fine to read for a while after you tuck yourself in, but essentially, reserve your bed for sleep, sex and sickness. If you do not sleep well one night, get up at the usual time anyway, stay active, and most likely you will sleep better the next night.

6. Get plenty of exercise during the day. The more energy you expend during the day, the sleepier you will feel at bedtime. It is important that the physical activity be earlier in the day as strenuous activity in the evening makes one alert and will impair sleep.
7. Reduce or eliminate your intake of stimulants such as caffeine (coffee, tea, cola, energy drinks, and chocolate). Even when consumed early in the day, these can impair sleep in susceptible people. When sleep is sufficient and refreshing, it is no longer necessary to have a cup of coffee in the morning in order to feel awake and alert. Cigarettes and alcohol can also impair sleep quality.
8. Avoid large meals late in the evening. Although one feels fatigued after a large festive meal, sleep is less restful and reflux is common.
9. Try a light evening snack, or the classic cup of warm milk, or a cup of caffeine-free tea—valerian root, chamomile, and peppermint are all good choices.

---

[74] Oats, rice, corn, ginger, barley and some nuts, seeds and vegetables contain melatonin. Tryptophan is an essential amino acid, which is a precursor for serotonin and melatonin. Foods high in tryptophan include: turkey, chicken, beef, game, fish, soybeans, spinach, brown rice, nuts, eggs, and dairy products. However, eating high protein foods results in the digestion of multiple amino acids, several of which compete with tryptophan for absorption into the brain. This is why consuming foods rich in complex carbohydrates (brown rice, nuts such as almonds, seeds, grains, fruits and vegetables) along with the protein source is a better way to increase your tryptophan absorption and aid in the production of serotonin, which helps to relax the body and improve sleep.

10. Add foods that contain melatonin or tryptophan to your evening meal.[74] 5-HTP (5-Hydroxytryptophan) is a naturally occurring amino acid that can increase levels of serotonin and melatonin in the brain. This supplement can be safely used to improve sleep.
11. Learn and practice a relaxation technique regularly. Breathing exercises, meditation, and prayer are good examples. When practised morning and evening, these activities can make you calmer and more relaxed and over time will improve sleep quality. The key is to quiet the mind as mental stillness will reduce intrusive thoughts from bubbling up into your consciousness.
12. While napping should not be necessary if you consistently get refreshing sleep, it is quite acceptable to have a short (15–30 minute) nap during the day—even more than once, if it makes you feel more alert. This is particularly important if you need to drive and you are feeling tired. Avoid long sleeps in the daytime, and avoid napping altogether if it interferes with your night sleep or if you suffer from insomnia.
13. Don't obsess if you can't sleep well occasionally. Learn to use your temporary insomnia as an opportunity to set goals, plan your day, to reflect on the things in life that you are thankful for or to just "be." Peaceful rest, when you are not able to sleep can be refreshing, especially if you use that time to go over your positive affirmations and practice relaxing breathing exercises (described in Habit Four: Be).
14. Cognitive-behavioral therapy (CBT) is the only scientifically proven non-drug treatment for insomnia.

CBT teaches you *how* to stop insomnia and is a natural insomnia remedy that has no side effects. There are several websites that offer CBT for insomnia.

15. Persistent insomnia may be due to a medical condition that can be treated. See a physician to rule out conditions such as heart failure, prostate enlargement, neurological conditions, as well as depression, anxiety, and obstructive sleep apnea (OSA). In addition, prescription medications, nicotine, caffeine, alcohol, and other substances can rob you of sleep.

Sleeplessness can result in weight gain, and obesity can lead to OSA. Beyond feeling un-refreshed in the morning, people who suffer from OSA are at increased risk of gastroesophageal reflux and heart disease. Often a dental device or surgical removal of the uvula at the back of the throat improves snoring and mild sleep apnea, but nasal CPAP (continuous positive airway pressure) therapy is required for severe sleep apnea. Many who suffer from OSA will get significant improvement when they lose weight.

# CHAPTER 10

*The most beautiful thing we can experience is the mysterious. It is the source of all true art and science.*

**Albert Einstein**

David had not yet finished reading his book but felt compelled to give Sanjay a call again to continue their conversation.

Sanjay thanked David for his interest in *12 Habits*. "I moved from India when I was seventeen. I planned on attending medical school, because I wanted to make a positive impact in the world," said the taxi driver by way of explanation. "Unfortunately, it didn't work out, so I had to find another means. That is why I founded the *Magna Vita Institute*: to help people find meaning and balance in their lives."

"Was it wholly altruistic, or did you also have a personal reason?" asked David. Sanjay was not at all fazed by the direct question. "I had been overweight and also had a family history of diabetes. I also knew that there was an epidemic of obesity and diabetes in North America and that I did not want to join that statistic. With the help of my family doctor and a local risk reduction clinic, I educated myself about nutrition and exercise."

"Although I knew that certain medications could reduce my risk of diabetes, I was determined to go as far as I could with lifestyle modifications alone," continued Sanjay. "I read a study that found that intensive lifestyle modifications trumped medication when it came to reducing risk of diabetes. It was a revelation to me."

"Interesting," said David. "I also have been doing a lot of reading, in my case about heart disease. Dietary and lifestyle choices seem to play a huge part in risk reduction. It sounds as if they are of equal importance in adult-onset diabetes."

> Diabetes due to insulin deficiency is termed Type 1 Diabetes Mellitus (DM). At this time there is nothing that can be done to prevent it (although some studies of diet in pregnancy and infancy are underway). Those who have Type 1 DM need to take insulin in addition to healthy lifestyle choices and control their blood sugars carefully to prevent complications. Type 2 Diabetes (T2DM) is mostly seen in overweight adults and does not initially require insulin. Many times, a low-GI diet and regular exercise resulting in weight loss are enough to control blood sugars. Often medications are needed and insulin may also be required if other treatments fail. T2DM is now seen in children and young adults as well because of the high incidence of childhood obesity.

Remembering his reading about eating whole foods while avoiding starchy foods with a high Glycemic Index, David asked Sanjay what his strategy was to lose weight as he had a genetic predisposition to diabetes.

"I tend to focus on raw nuts and seeds," said Sanjay. "Since a seed contains all the building blocks to grow a whole plant—they are bound to be very nutritious."

"I have read about the importance of the essential fatty acids that are found in oily nuts and seeds, but I haven't really focused on them yet," replied David.

"Let me tell you a story about one of my favourite seeds. You remember the 'Chia Pet,' don't you?" asked Sanjay.

"Yes, a clay figure of a head or animal on which you applied chia seeds. After regular watering, they sprout into green 'hair' or 'fur,'" responded David.

"Well, that very seed was prized by the Aztecs who carried sacks of it with them when going on long voyages. As little as one tablespoon of seeds a day with plenty of water was enough to sustain them," enthused Sanjay. "Chia seeds are the most hydrophilic (water absorbing) food known. A mixture of one part seed with ten parts water makes a gel that can be used to replace fats when baking. The soluble and insoluble fibres make the seeds filling and excellent for intestinal regularity. Like other oily seeds, they are a good source of essential fatty acids as well as minerals and protein."

"I will definitely find ways to add chia seeds to my diet," David told him, "just as I did quinoa! Did you know," he asked Sanjay, "that quinoa is a grain that contains all the essential amino acids required for human nutrition, making it a complete protein—much like meats? I like its texture and flavour and it's a great substitute for rice, pasta, or potatoes."

Sanjay laughed. "You've really been doing your research, David! I knew soya beans were a good source of protein but now I'll add quinoa into my recipes."

David was planning to work out that afternoon and Sanjay needed to start his shift in the taxi. They agreed to meet again soon. As David cycled to the Peninsula Club, he continued to think about the many ways in which diet can influence health.

He recalled that at his last appointment, Osler had mentioned a study that showed that the "phagocytic index" of white blood cells is suppressed for six hours after a sugar load. This refers to the ability of the cells to engulf viral and bacterial particles and thereby neutralize them.

"That is, white blood cells (an important part of the immune system) are not able to do their job when we take in a diet high in sugar," Osler had said, sensing David's interest in the subject. "I think that is why children who consume a lot of candy, pop, and other sweet snacks are more likely to catch colds than other kids. I don't think it is only the virus. Remember that all the kids in a classroom are exposed to the same virus, but some get sick all the time, and others never do. A robust immune system makes all the difference—and I think that nutrition, sleep, and exercise influence that significantly."

As he neared the club, David thought guiltily of the "treats" that he had previously insisted on purchasing for Adam and Rebecca and was determined to think of wiser alternatives. He and Jessica had frequently quarrelled about the importance of feeding the kids healthy meals and snacks. She had always gone to a lot of effort to prepare fresh, wholesome meals for her family, and he now realized that he had been sabotaging that effort. He remembered with a smile how Jessica had threatened to take the kids to a greasy burger joint if they brought home a poor report card! He, on the other hand, had felt that taking the kids to popular restaurants for fast food was a treat for them. "Why would I treat my kids with crappy food? What was I thinking?" he asked himself out loud.

Recalling how pleased the whole family had been with his culinary skill on the evening of the salmon barbeque, he resolved that he would build on that experience to support Jessica in raising healthy children.

David had taken up the saxophone with great gusto in his high school band but had given it up once he got to the university. He had kept his instrument, but had somehow never managed to get back to playing. Now, with unexpected time on his hands, he retrieved it from his apartment closet, and started to play once more. Rusty though he was, David could tell that he was not just mechanically belting out tunes, but that the music itself was starting to flow through him. As he played more regularly, he realized that at the age of forty-two, all of his life experiences, including his separation from Jessica, his recent health crisis, and his new-found interest in changing his lifestyle, were being poured into his musical expression.

*Where the spirit does not work with the hand there is no art.*

**Leonardo Da Vinci** (1452–1519) Italian artist, architect, musician, inventor, and scientist.[75]

**HABIT NINE: INDULGE IN THE ARTS**

When visiting a city or when needing to take a break from one's usual activities, a trip to a museum, art gallery, or park is a great way to refresh oneself. Connecting with nature and the arts not only reduces stress, but inspires us to be more creative. See plays or other theatrical productions regularly and support your local symphony orchestra or other musical groups.

"Sixty years and twenty minutes," was the way late Canadian painter Toni Onley described how long it took him to produce a painting. He used a unique blend of West Coast Modernism with traditional oriental brush techniques to creative distinctive watercolour

[75] Gelb, Michael, 1998. *How to Think Like Leonardo da Vinci: Seven Steps to Genius Every Day*, Dell Trade Paperback, Dell Publishing, a division of Random House, New York, New York. Da Vinci designed bridges and aqueducts, flying machines, parachutes, submarines, underwater breathing devices, and even contact lenses. His knowledge of the human form led to the creation of the first anatomy textbook. Gelb gives strategies to tap into this kind of creative genius.

landscapes. These paintings would flow through him swiftly and effortlessly as he painted at remote locations, yet were clearly the culmination of his life's experiences and training.

**One minute message**

Optimum health requires use of both sides of the brain. The *left brain* is logical, analytical, and objective; the *right brain* is intuitive, holistic, and subjective. The *arts* allow us to bridge the *left* and the *right hemispheres*.

Challenge yourself to be creative: learn to play an instrument, learn a new language, sing in a choir, take an art class or cooking class.

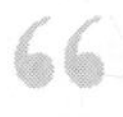

Visual artists can be either painters or sculptors. Painters add colour and form to a canvas to create beauty. The sculptor can also create beauty by building objects out of metal, wood, or other material. But carvers and sculptors also chip away things to reveal the beauty hidden within. The "Slaves" of Michelangelo are unfinished sculptures that reveal the creative process of how the figures are encased in marble that needs to be removed in order to reveal them. Michelangelo said that he didn't sculpt figures into marble: he liberated them out of it. He quarried his own marble in Carrara, seeing the finished sculptures in the living rock before driving in the first nail that would split it off the rock face. The unfinished slaves are deeply compelling examples of how Michelangelo chipped away the marble enclosure, gradually exposing more and more of the figures trapped inside.

Inasmuch as life imitates art, this difference can be seen in our lives as well. Beauty and success can be achieved by adding things to what already exists—adding knowledge and skill to shape one's talents, for example taking a cooking or painting class, doing woodworking, or training for medical and surgical specialties. Conversely, less desirable attributes, habits, addictions, and personality traits that stand in the way of success can be identified and eliminated to allow a person to achieve his or her full potential. Many times, both techniques are necessary. As we have discussed earlier, to achieve optimum health, the same steps are necessary; it is important to embrace good habits of nutritious eating, exercise, and rest, while at the same time eliminating the harmful habits that create barriers to good health.

"What's the best way of dropping habits that harm our health?" asked David on his next visit to Dr. Osler.

"By identifying them and taking strategic steps to improve them. Sometimes that can happen serendipitously. Let me tell you the story of my colleague, Dr. Robert James." replied Osler. "Rob is a family practice doc in White Rock, British Columbia who's been in practice for over twenty-five years. Over the years managed to pack on about forty pounds of excess weight. He started doing something about it quite by accident. One week, his wife, Jane was away at a conference, and he was running late for the office. He looked in the fridge and found a container of cottage cheese. He decided to have a few spoonfuls before rushing off. He ended up working through his lunch hour as he needed to see a couple of patients in the hospital, and by the time he got home he was too tired to prepare a big meal, so he foraged salad greens, tomatoes, and cucumbers from the fridge. The next morning, he realized that he had not eaten a lot of carbs the previous day. For the sake of experiment, he decided to limit his breakfast to a cup of yogurt. He had a small tin of tuna at lunch and another salad in the evening. He did make a point of drinking at least six glasses of water a day."

"By the time Jane got home Rob was on a roll. He told her that he was on a 'zero carbohydrate diet' and feeling great! He had lost five pounds in that first week and continued more or less the same pattern for the next two months by which time he had trimmed thirty-five pounds from his torso. *This is not so hard*, he thought, *so why can't more people do it?* He told all his overweight patients about his 'zero carb' diet and that if he could do it so could they. He argued that all you need is a little protein to maintain your muscles and neurotransmitters, a fair bit of roughage to promote good evacuation of the colon, and water for hydration. He felt one did not need to take a lot of supplements or spend money on complicated cleanses because everything you need can be provided in your diet—as long as you make the point of taking in what you need and strictly avoiding what you don't need."

"The reality was that Rob was eating far less than before and his weight loss could be entirely attributed to caloric restriction. It was not a magical diet but simply less food. A recent study demonstrated that it did not matter what kind of diet subjects followed; when calories were restricted and exercise was increased, weight loss occurred.

**Four diets were compared:**

1. 20% fat, 15% protein, 65% carbohydrate (low fat)
2. 20% fat, 25% protein, 55% carbohydrate (high protein)
3. 40% fat, 15% protein, 45% carbohydrate (high fat)
4. 40% fat, 25% protein, 35% carbohydrate (low carb)

All diets were balanced by dieticians to ensure that healthy fats were used, and that all participants received plenty of fruits, vegetables, and whole grains. Each participant was counselled to reduce calories by 750 per day, and to exercise a minimum of ninety minutes a week. Perhaps not surprisingly, weight loss and risk reduction were similar in all groups. The study concluded that any diet taught with enthusiasm and persistence can be effective for weight loss as well as cardiovascular and diabetic risk reduction. Diets can be tailored to individuals based on personal and cultural preferences to have the best chance of long-term success."[76]

........................................................................

David had not been to one of Adam's soccer games for a few weeks, so he made an effort to go this Saturday despite the pouring rain. He felt bad that he had not made the time to contribute more to the team, as he had volunteered to be assistant coach. He spoke to the coach, Justin, after the game to congratulate him on what he had

---

[76] Sacks et al., 2009, Comparison of Weight-Loss Diets with Different Compositions of Fat, Protein, and Carbohydrates, *New England Journal of Medicine*. Vol. 360 No. 9 Feb 26. This well designed two-year study compared various levels of macronutrients while using similar caloric restriction. Each participant had the same caloric deficit (total energy was approximately 2000 calories in each group). Each group received the same exercise recommendation and behavioural counselling. Despite great variation in the amount of fats, proteins and carbohydrates, all groups had a similar weight loss and reduction in cardiovascular and diabetic risk.

accomplished with the team this year. "How did you find the time to commit to a practice and a game each week?" asked David sheepishly.

"Hey David, I'm happy to see you whenever you are able to make it out to a practice or game. I fully understand that you are maxed out in your law practice and that you are now recovering from your heart attack. The last thing you need is more stress and deadlines—trust me, I can handle these boys! Besides, I love to play soccer myself and want to help my son Matthias and the others to develop their skills and learn the importance of working as a team," replied Justin. "Some of the boys may not be able to afford to go to college but a sports scholarship might give them that opportunity," he added. Justin also admitted that the warm up and training exercises he did with the team were pretty much the only exercise he was getting lately. "So this way I get to multi-task."

"Time is always a consideration," continued Justin. "There's just not enough of it. So I try to stay active by taking the stairs at work, parking a block or two from my destinations, and sitting on an exercise ball instead of the sofa while I watch a movie or a game on TV. My dad has a novel approach," he continued. "When he reads, often for two or three hours a day, he never does so while relaxing on a comfortable chair. Instead, he lays belly down on a stool or dining room chair, with his legs held out straight behind him, strengthening his core and back muscles while reading his book in front of him on the floor."

*What a great example of Incidental Exercise, described in Habit Two*, thought David.

As the team was packing up after their game, some of

the boys asked if they could go to Splendour Blender for a power shake to refuel. David said he would meet them there; he needed to pick up Rebecca from her riding lesson. Adam had been hoping to hang out a bit more with Matthias and his other teammates and asked if he could catch a ride with Justin.

David drove out on his own to Campbell Valley, an area dotted by magnificent equestrian estates and a few riding stables. Rebecca had finished her lesson and was brushing her horse when her father arrived. He stood quietly for a few minutes watching her, incredibly proud of how his daughter was already so responsible and determined at her young age.

When she looked up and saw her father, Rebecca gave him a big smile and threw her arms around him. "I love you, Daddy." After she finished cleaning up, they both thanked the riding instructor and drove off to join Adam and his team.

It was a misty but beautiful day on the rolling country roads and David was savouring the one-on-one time with his precious daughter. She excitedly told him that today she got to ride Patriot; she was the youngest student ever to be trusted with this majestic chestnut stallion! David was taking in the landscape and glancing at his happy child while still watching the road carefully. As they crested a small hill he saw a car coming directly towards them on the wrong side of the road. He swerved right to avoid a head-on collision, but the car struck them hard near the rear door on the driver's side and spun them around. David managed to avoid a power pole but still ended up in the ditch beside the road. The passenger window smashed and he heard Rebecca scream in pain.

David, who felt a searing pain in the back of his neck and between his shoulder blades, realized his hands were numb and tingling. However, he was able to move his arms and legs, and so he undid his seat belt. Rebecca was still securely belted and her air bag had deployed. Her face had multiple small glass cuts and her right forearm was bleeding from a puncture wound. David used his cell phone to call 911, praying that the ambulance would arrive quickly. He opened Rebecca's seatbelt and saw that her arm was obviously deformed. He would not be able to get her out the passenger side so he carefully extricated her through his door. Rebecca seemed otherwise uninjured and sat down at the side of the road supporting her right arm. David went to check out the other vehicle. Still running, its front end was smashed in. The driver, a woman in her mid-fifties who reeked of alcohol and stale smoke, was slumped over the wheel. She had a laceration on her forehead but was conscious. David turned the motor off and told the woman that an ambulance was on its way. Then he dashed back to Rebecca.

The paramedics checked out Rebecca first and applied a splint to her arm. A piece of bone had poked through the skin, indicating that this was an open fracture contaminated with skin bacteria and would need to be cleaned and repaired in the operating room. Rebecca and David were taken to the hospital in the ambulance while a tow truck was called for David's damaged car. A second ambulance soon arrived to transport the driver of the other vehicle to hospital.

Jessica, who had received a call from David, met them at the hospital. She had picked up Adam, explained the situation to him, and left him with her parents before making the trip to the hospital. She gave David a sideways glance; she knew that David loved his kids but he had now been in two major accidents in the last month, and although she knew neither was his fault she was regretting her decision to let him pick their daughter up.

Rebecca had x-rays taken and was seen by the orthopedic surgeon on call. Dr. Salter advised them that he would need to operate on Rebecca's arm to clean the wound and align the bone, using a metal plate with screws to hold the broken bone in place. He went over the usual risks of surgery—bleeding, infection, inadvertent injury to surrounding structures, as well as possible anaesthetic risks, but stated that these risks were small, and that she absolutely required the operation to have a functional arm again. David and Jessica consented to the surgery and waited anxiously for the doctor to emerge from the OR.

Dr. Salter returned later and told them the operation had gone well. He stated that the fracture was fixed and should heal just fine. He did not feel that the injury would result in any long-term disability. One of her parents could stay with her at all times as Rebecca would need to remain in the hospital for IV antibiotics for a day or two.

After four days in the hospital, Rebecca developed a high fever and her wound was discharging. Cultures were done, which showed that she had picked up a hospital-acquired "staph infection" that was resistant to multiple medications. Rebecca was transferred to the ICU and started on stronger antibiotics. Unfortunately, she did not respond to the antibiotics, so she was taken back to the OR to have the wound reopened and the infected tissue dissected out. To the incredulity of her parents, Rebecca's condition continued to deteriorate. She became septic, slipped into a coma, and began having seizures.

Jessica and David were united in their outrage and fear. Their daughter had suffered a serious fracture that required surgery, but this was an injury that was well within the scope of their local hospital to repair. They had not remotely considered that Rebecca would develop a serious complication and be left fighting for her life.

The girl was transferred to the regional Children's Hospital, where she was intubated and mechanically ventilated. She received intensive therapy with antibiotics and medications to support her blood pressure. She was chilled with ice packs and cold IV infusions to lower her temperature to a hypothermic level. It was hoped that these heroic measures would conserve her healing energy and protect her brain, as there was concern that the coma and seizures might have resulted in reduced oxygen getting to her brain.

David and Jessica spent most of their time in Rebecca's room together. They asked her doctor what the realistic chances were of Rebecca recovering.

"Everything that can be done is being done. Take it day by day," said Dr. Ward pragmatically. "Hold Rebecca's hand, talk to her, and on some level she will know you are there. The best you can do in these circumstances is hope and pray she will hear you and get better."

To David and Jessica that did not sound like there was much that they could contribute to their daughter's recovery but took that advice to heart and clung to it. The crisis brought the pair closer again. They stayed with Rebecca around the clock and took turns reading to her, singing to her, and praying with her. When friends called and asked what they could do to help, David and Jessica repeated their mantra; "Just hope and pray—hope and pray."

Rebecca's condition stabilized somewhat and she seemed to be trying to breathe again. Dr. Ward turned the settings on the machine down to see if they might be able to pull out the tube and let Rebecca breathe on her own. She opened her eyes briefly, and it looked as if she was smiling at her parents. Dr. Ward turned the ventilator down. But it was too soon: Rebecca was not able to breathe by herself. He was able to reduce her meds, but she was still in a coma and required mechanical ventilation.

A few more agonizing days dragged by. They knew that the longer she remained unresponsive, the greater the risk that she would be left with significant impairments—if she made it at all. With each passing hour, their hope faded a little more. They spoke to the social worker and the transplant team about organ donation—enabling Rebecca to give the gift of life to some other unfortunate people. They were surprised to learn how many body parts could be harvested and transplanted so that perhaps a half-a-dozen lives could be saved and at least another half-dozen lives improved. They discussed how her heart and lungs, kidneys, liver, pancreas, pituitary, corneas, parts of her intestine, bones, bone marrow, and even tendons could live on in others. It was a noble but macabre discussion. David and Jessica liked the idea that Rebecca would able to save lives and restore vision, but could not bear the thought of losing their daughter. They remembered her dreams of becoming a teacher and a riding instructor when she grew up, and could not accept that her life was holding on by a thread.

On Easter Sunday, Jessica brought Adam to the hospital to see his sister. Rebecca opened her eyes as they entered her room. She tried to cough. The ICU nurse came over as

Rebecca was trying to pull her tube out. The nurse turned down the ventilator settings and gave Rebecca a mild sedative, as she was fighting the breathing machine. She paged the on-call doctor. When he arrived, he turned the ventilator down further, and Rebecca continued to breathe on her own. A few minutes later, he extubated her, and she began to cough. She opened her eyes and smiled.

"Welcome back, Becca! Happy Easter," said Adam.

Rebecca was transferred to the step-down unit on the following day. She had a deep scar but her wound healed. To her parents' utter relief, Rebecca suffered no neurological damage and was as bright and charming as she was prior to the accident. David and Jessica were not particularly religious, yet the coincidence of their daughter rising again on Easter morning was not lost on them. A month later, Rebecca needed one more operation to reposition some of the muscles and tendons that had been severed when her infected wound was debrided. She went on to make a complete recovery.

The accident provided many painful lessons. The driver who had hit David's car had two previous charges of impaired driving and had a suspended license; she should not have even been on the road. The operation that Rebecca underwent was fairly routine; she should have made an uneventful recovery—but hospital-acquired infections, as Jessica and David learnt, are shockingly common. A short time later, David visited Dr. Osler and shared the story of the senseless accident, the life threatening infection, and the miraculous recovery.

Osler told David that he had served on the Safety and Quality Committee of St. Luke's. "I found it difficult but important to conduct quality reviews of bad outcomes, as it gave the hospital an opportunity to look at the whole healthcare system, not blaming an individual, but trying to make global changes to improve the system that everyone works in. Every system is perfectly designed to achieve the results that it gets, and if you put good people into a poor system, the system will beat them every time."[77]

"Medical errors are somewhat difficult to track but include preventable events such as a huge variety of medication errors, diagnostic and radiological tests being misinterpreted, wrong site or inappropriate surgery, serious complications, falls and injuries, and hospital acquired infections," continued Osler in a reflective mood. "It has been estimated that there are well over one million medication errors a year in the United States alone. Deaths from medical errors are so prevalent that they may account for the third most common cause of death—right after heart disease and cancer. They are not well publicized, but to put it into perspective, it would be equivalent to more than two jumbo-jets crashing every week.[78] And the United States is not alone with regard to medical errors: the statistics are comparable in a number of countries including Canada, Australia, and several European nations."

"Why do bright, well-trained and compassionate health-care givers make so many errors?" asked David.

---

[77] The Institute for Healthcare Improvement (IHI) was founded in the 1980s by Dr. Donald Berwick, and other visionaries. This health-care quality and safety organization based in Boston, Massachusetts, is dedicated to measuring and improving health outcomes and saving hundreds of thousands of lives by implementing numerous patient safety strategies. IHI is committed to improving health care *systems* in order to improve health outcomes. In July 2010, President Obama appointed Dr. Berwick as the new administrator of the Centers for Medicare & Medicaid Services.

[78] Starfield, Barbara, 2000, Is US Health really the Best in the World? *The Journal of the American Medical Association (JAMA)* Vol .284, No 4, July 26th. Medical errors may account for up to 100,000 deaths a year in America.

"There are many reasons for this as healthcare is such a complex system. Toxic solutions and medications are being administered, and it is easy to give a wrong med or a wrong dosage or to give the medication to the wrong patient," replied Osler. "By the way, errors do not include those instances when the right meds are given to the right patient in the correct dose and a bad outcome results, as adverse effects are known to occur. The potential for such adverse side effects must be weighed in the prescribing process."

"The healthcare system is so large and multifaceted that sufficient checks and balances are not always possible, especially in emergency situations. Caregiver fatigue is often a factor. Contaminated substances may not be properly disposed of, making infection more likely. Hygiene and infection control may not be optimal. Sometimes the left and right limb—or a patient name—may be mixed up. At times there may an error in judgment."

"Systems can and have been put in place to mitigate medical errors. However, unanticipated events will continue to occur as 'the holes in the Swiss cheese' line up. A series of almost inconsequential slips by skilled and benevolent caregivers often happen simultaneously and combine to cause a tragedy."[79]

"Medical errors are taking an unacceptably high toll on our society, while healthcare costs are spiralling out of control and can no longer be sustained. Radical and innovative solutions need to be sought to make healthcare safer and affordable. This includes more health education with emphasis on prevention

---

[79] Gladwell, Malcolm, 2008, To better understand how an accumulation of minor difficulties and malfunctions cause most catastrophic accidents, *see Outliers*, Little, Brown and Company, New York, pages 182–184.

[80] Goldhill, David, 2009, How American Health Care Killed My Father, *The Atlantic*, Sept.

and self-care as well as new funding models that introduce free market concepts of competition and accountability and set standards for quality and safety,"[80] concluded Osler.

# CHAPTER 11

*Man, alone, has the power to transform his thoughts into physical reality; man, alone, can dream and make his dreams come true.*

**Napoleon Hill**
(1883–1970) American author whose best-known work is Think and Grow Rich.

After the crisis of Rebecca's injury had subsided, David called Sanjay to ask if they could meet for tea. Although his daughter was recovering well, David woke up each morning with his stomach in knots. His head often ached and for no apparent reason he felt tired and lightheaded. At times his fingers felt numb and tingled.

Sanjay was a sympathetic listener. "Stress can make you physically sick. This may be why walking outside in the winter with a tee shirt and wet hair can actually give you a cold. Believing that a treatment will help you increases the likelihood that it will. Believing that a medication will give you a side effect increases that probability as well. The immune system can be conditioned like Pavlov's dogs, such that a physical cue (taste, sound, or image) can stimulate healing or illness!"[81]

David sat mesmerized as he listened to Sanjay. "Now, I'm not a doctor," Sanjay went on, "but it has always been fascinating to me that a positive attitude can make all the difference. When things are going well in life, good things happen, and when things go wrong, we start to spiral downwards. Like begets like, as they say. When I became interested in how the mind affects the body and the body affects the mind, I started reading a lot about it and attending conferences. 'Mind Body Medicine' is a huge field that includes therapies such as guided imagery, biofeedback, energetic healing, and hypnotherapy. And think about the 'placebo effect.' This response (from the Latin 'to please') is a positive outcome following the

---

[81] Azar, Beth, 2001. A New Take On Psychoneuroimmunology. Research pointing to a circuit linking the immune system and brain connects illness, stress, mood, and thought in a whole new way. *Monitor on Psychology, Journal of the American Psychological Association,* December, Vol 32, No. 11, page 34

administration of an inert substance. This response needs to be accounted for in clinical trials as it is known that giving any substance will result in a positive effect in some people. Hence, 'placebo controlled trials' have an inactive placebo group and an active treatment group."

The opposite effect is a 'nocebo' response (Latin 'I shall harm') where a harmless substance results in a negative outcome—think of a voodoo doll. Physicians need to be careful to avoid 'medical hexing' as well; when an authoritative doctor with a white coat tells a patient he only has three months to live—the patient may comply and die as predicted."

"More recently, a lot of this thinking converged to create the science known as psychoneuroimmunology.[82] What a mouthful that word is! This is the study of how emotions and the mind influence health through connections between the nervous system, hormone system and the immune system. Now that the human genome has been mapped out, a great deal of chromosomal research is going on. It turns out that emotional signals can influence which genes are expressed and therefore which proteins and messengers they produce. In other words, the chromosomal blueprint is fixed—but what we build from the blueprint can be influenced!"

Sanjay paused. Seeing that David was intrigued by this subject, he continued. "It has long been understood that stress causes a release of hormones from the brain and adrenal glands, which can raise blood pressure and heart rate, make us feel shaky, sweaty, and anxious—and it can increase

---

[82] Ader, Robert coined the term *Psychoneuroimmunology* in 1975 to describe the scientific field of study investigating the bi-directional communications among the nervous system, the endocrine (hormone) system, and the immune system, and the implications of these linkages for physical health.

our risk of heart disease. The really cool thing now is that there is scientific proof that our thoughts can influence our DNA! It has been demonstrated that the expression of more than a thousand genes can be influenced by meditation. Regularly practising relaxation breathing exercises results in more genes being expressed that reduce inflammation throughout the body as well as lower blood pressure."

"Hmmm, that sounds like some trendy new-age science," ventured David.

"Well, in fact, the earliest reference I found recognizing the mind-body connection was attributed to Hippocrates, who in about 400 BC lamented that the great error of his day was that physicians separate the soul from the body!" replied Sanjay.

"So how do we use this information to improve our health?" David's curiosity was piqued.

"Being aware is the first step. Letting go of negative thoughts and emotions and avoiding the free fall into despair when things go wrong. Too often when we suffer a disappointment we tend to generalize that life is all bad. We need to see setbacks in perspective, learn from them, and move on. At the same time, we need to believe that good things will be drawn to us. Surrounding ourselves with optimistic people and joyful attitudes will help manifest greatness into our lives. When someone asks me how I am, I usually say 'tremendous,' as it starts to get some positive juices flowing!"

"Having the knowledge and insight that emotions and beliefs influence health and other outcomes is the most important step. Next steps include practising those skills—visualize clearly what you want, then develop a detailed step-by-step strategy of how you will achieve it—then have the confidence to reach your goal."

Sanjay's infectious enthusiasm impressed David, despite his initial scepticism. He agreed to give it a try. After all, he had never been afraid to try something new—especially if it was something that could be so powerful and effective. He remembered what he had read about making positive affirmations in his *12 Habits* booklet. Sanjay's discussion had just shed some light on how affirmations work.

*The greater danger for most of us lies not in setting our aim too high and falling short; but in setting our aim too low and achieving our mark.*

**Michelangelo** (1475–1564) Born in Florence, Italy, Michelangelo Buonarroti's art mirrored his belief that the beauty of the human body was a symbol of divinity.

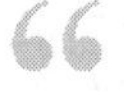

**HABIT TEN: LIFELONG LEARNING**

One of the most important things we can do is to remain curious. For example, learning new languages can help us to communicate better when we travel or speak with people from different countries. This process can result in a deeper understanding of a culture and people, and it can also help to form new neural pathways in the brain, which keeps us mentally sharp and slows the aging process.

**One minute message**

Neural connections that allow us to learn new information are most abundant in childhood and wither away as we age.

*Learning* new information helps keep our minds sharp and delays the *aging process*. It is also the only way to stay current in our professional lives as well as to satisfy our curiosities in fields that may be familiar or foreign.

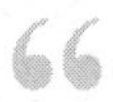

Learning a musical instrument or singing in a choir also brings joy and satisfaction to both the listener as well as the musician. Not only is one filled with a sense of accomplishment and wellbeing after a good practice or performance, but it may also make us more resilient to illness. Mozart's final composition was the *Requiem*, which contains the hauntingly beautiful prayer "Lacrimosa." Blood tests done on choir members who sang Mozart's "Lacrimosa" were found to have elevated levels of immunopeptides after a performance. This elevation was not evident in members of the audience used as controls. This indicates that the act of singing can boost one's immune system and possibly promote healing!

There are unlimited opportunities to learn specific new skills and techniques. In addition to learning languages and practising music, one can explore a vast array of historical and academic pursuits, travel, culinary options, arts, crafts, and specialized training in professional fields. You are never really too old to learn something new, or even to make a significant career or life change. It may require some courage and faith, however. Take for example Father Maurice "Moe" Schroder (1937–) who was asked how he felt about being nearly forty before becoming a physician. Fr. Moe replied that he would be forty whether he were practising medicine or not!

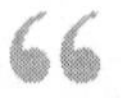

Maurice Schroder is a Canadian from Saskatchewan who was ordained a Roman Catholic priest in 1962 and joined the Oblate Order. He wanted to do medical missionary work, so he enrolled in the medical school at the University of Calgary in 1969. Since 1978, Fr. Moe has been serving the indigenous people of the Amazon Basin in Peru. He was joined by Fr. Jack MacCarthy, an American from Wisconsin, who was ordained a Norbertine priest in 1969. He studied medicine at Loyola University Medical School in Chicago, graduating in 1977. Fr. Jack then completed an Internal Medicine residency in Minnesota, and learned Spanish. He was medical director of a tropical medicine clinic on the Island of St. Lucia in the West Indies before joining Fr. Moe at the isolated Santa Clotilde clinic in Peru in 1985. The two physician-priests run a forty-bed mission hospital there and also service twelve remote outposts along the rivers.[83] Not to be ignored in the quest for knowledge is the cognitive and spiritual work that will move us closer to optimal health and happiness. This includes some of the techniques on meditation and relaxation discussed in Habit 4—Be, as well as Habit 6—Spiritual Awareness. These are all positive things to learn and to

[83] Fr. Moe and Fr. Jack were in Vancouver, Canada in September 2010 where the author had the opportunity to meet them. They are dedicated healers who work long hours and fully devote themselves to their combined ministries of Serving the Soul and Healing the Body. Fr. Moe spoke of their mission work as being "inter-faith." He explained that no matter what faith group, if any, you belonged to, be it Christian, Jewish, or Atheist, the only thing that mattered was the genuine desire to serve those in need. They were setting up a non-governmental organization (NGO) to support their work at Centro de Salud Santa Clotilde in the spirit of one of the author's colleagues, the late Dr. Kerry Telford-Morrissey, a Vancouver family physician, who had gone to Peru four times as a physician volunteer. Along with her infant daughter, Sarah, Kerry died in a sea plane accident in British Columbia on November 29, 2009.

practise. Lifelong learning also involves a certain "letting go" of negative influences. Some of these were discussed in Habit 3—Out with the Bad—which focused mainly on substances such as tobacco smoke that stands in the way of wellness, or environmental toxins that sabotage health and promote illness. However, other more insidious barriers to good health are negative emotions. These may be notoriously difficult to identify and control, yet undoubtedly contribute to the stress and anxiety that we feel. Unchecked, they lead to unhappiness and contribute to ill being. Harbouring feelings of anger, hatred, jealousy, and resentment can have devastating effects on the people around us, but are also a poison that erodes the vessel that bears them. Anger is like hot coal; it burns those who hold it. In the words of the Buddha—Siddhartha Gautama (c. 653 BC) — "You will not be punished for your anger—you will be punished by your anger."

Becoming proficient with the sax was giving David a lot of joy. He was not only playing by himself but he had recently joined a jazz sextet. The keyboard player was a gifted young man named Carl Bray from Saskatchewan who had studied music in Toronto, Ontario. In his first year of study, Carl had won the prestigious Oscar Peterson Scholarship offered annually to only one jazz student in Canada. David felt more than a little out of his league playing with this group; other than the bassist, who was a senior music teacher, he was also the eldest—however he enjoyed the challenge as it made him stretch his capabilities. He had known about Carl Bray's abilities and dreamed that one day he might be able to play with him … now it was a reality! In fact, when they had the opportunity to play a concert together on the big stage at a jazz festival in Vancouver, David got such a euphoric feeling that he would later tell his friends it was the most fun he had ever had with his clothes on!

Sanjay attended the gig. Afterwards, over a glass of wine, David talked at length about his love for jazz. "Although there are rules to follow and a specific melody and key, it is more free-flowing than classical music or rock, and provides a unique opportunity to improvise."

"As a teenager, I liked to noodle on the guitar and sax, playing whatever came into my head." said David. "I never really liked the Royal Conservatory approach to music teaching; I thought it stifled creativity and innovation."

Sanjay agreed that music as well as sports should never lose sight of being fun. "Kids are enrolled in sports for fitness and fun and to learn the skills of sportsmanship and team play and competition, but too often, parents and coaches take it far too seriously and thereby take out the joy that brought the kids there in the first place."

"I find this not only to be the case in sports, but organizing or institutionalizing anything runs the risk of spoiling the underlying pursuit for which that institution was created," continued Sanjay. "I could give you examples from fields as diverse as farming practices, marriage, religion, education, and health care. For instance, the commercialization of food production can reduce the nutritional content, disconnect consumers from their food, and have grave consequences on the environment that is needed to grow the food in the first place."

"However, food can be nourishing to our bodies and

minds and does not need to deplete the land, soil, water, and other resources needed to produce it. Growing small gardens, supporting local farmers' markets and organic producers are steps in the direction of sustainability," summed up Sanjay.

"You're a wise man, Sanjay," said David. "It's meant a lot to me to work through 12 Habits and to incorporate the ideas and habits into my life. Meditation does not come easily, however."

"With patience and practice it is possible to achieve conscious awareness without thinking of anything in particular," replied Sanjay simply. "It's about the ability of setting the brain on 'receive'... being open and attentive to incoming information without trying to control it. Remarkable insights can occur in this way."

"I encourage you, David, to practise being present in the moment. When you are speaking to your kids, be fully present at that time. Gently brush aside distracting thoughts. When speaking to clients, co-workers, or friends, give these people your full attention and concentration. This also helps us to remember what was spoken. When you are walking by yourself, remain in the moment. Thinking about stresses from the past or challenges of the future does not alter those events; it only robs you of the joy of being present in the moment you are living now! By choosing to live mindfully in the moment you will be more aware of the beauty of things around you and derive more meaning from conversations and interactions you have."

..........

At his next medical appointment, David reviewed his cardiac status with Dr. Osler. His blood pressure was good, his cholesterol level was well controlled, and he was eating better, exercising more, and learning coping and stress-reduction techniques. "I understand the fundamentals of nutrition a lot better now, but I feel I need a more structured plan to get rid of twenty excess pounds," said David.

"Fundamentally, healthy eating is not about restricting food intake," Dr. Osler began. "It's really about eating sensible portions of nutritious foods. The more healthy foods we put on our plates, the more that crowds out the less healthy choices. Having said that, there are some specific guidelines I can suggest to help you reach your goal. I often give my patients tips for losing weight by simply creating a caloric deficit—consume fewer calories and burn more," Osler continued. "This seems obvious, but is surprisingly challenging for many people to do. I'm very much against any 'quick fix diet,' as it is temporary and therefore unsustainable. Furthermore, I don't like the idea of leaving certain healthy foods out of the diet for the purpose of losing weight."

> Setting SMART goals: They must be Specific, Measureable, Achievable, Resourced, and Timed. Specific goals may be to walk fifteen minutes three times per week, or to consume no more than 1600 calories a day, or no calories will be consumed after 7:00 PM. Measurable means counting calories, pounds, abdominal circumference, miles, or time. Achievable is realistic; it may not be possible to lose twenty pounds in a month or to run a marathon with three months of training. Resourced refers to the things you need to accomplish your goal. Make sure you have a good pair of running shoes, access to a bike, a calorie counter, heart rate monitor, and so forth. Timed refers to how long it should reasonably take to achieve the goal.

"More often than not, patients try one fad diet after the other, regain any weight they may have lost and learn nothing about nutrition. I much prefer to problem-solve around various weight loss strategies in order to help my patients reach their goals."

"One thing I have found effective is to give my patients something unambiguous. It is somewhat prescriptive, but then I prescribe medications all the time, too," said the doctor with a grin. "I've prepared a short handout that I call 'The Osler Diet.' This is my version of a heart-smart diet that is also effective for weight loss. The diet consists of three phases: an initial restrictive phase to reduce calories and challenge the dieter to try new options; a second less restrictive phase, still designed to lose weight; and a third, sensible maintenance phase. Here's your copy, David. Give it a whirl."

## THE OSLER DIET

**PHASE ONE:** This phase is very low in processed carbohydrates. Do your best to avoid all high GI foods. By eliminating all foods high in sugar and refined carbohydrates (flour) for two weeks, four things start to happen. Firstly, weight starts to drop simply because less is being eaten. Secondly, the caloric restriction results in the burning of stored body fat. Thirdly, the dieter looks for healthier alternatives. Finally (and most importantly) the dieter feels better—more energetic. The person may also feel a sense of satisfaction in having accomplished the two-week goal—and he or she may start getting positive feedback for sticking to the plan and already looking slimmer.

As is the case with many things in life, achieving a great outcome requires some hard work and sacrifice. If someone is not willing to cut back on comfort foods or even staples in their diet for two weeks, for the sake of better health and feeling more energetic, they simply lack the motivation and determination required to make meaningful lifestyle changes. In that case, they must suffer the consequences of obesity or work with their physicians to optimize their medications, consider weight loss surgery, or otherwise put their trust in the hands of the healthcare system. If, on the other hand, someone is motivated to do what they can to improve their health and reduce their medications, aggressive dietary changes for two short weeks are easily achievable.

Many cultures and religions promote periods of fasting or abstinence from certain foods to encourage self-denial, deepen gratitude for what we have, strengthen spiritual connections, and to create savings that can be invested in worthwhile charities. At the same time, many practitioners of natural medicine promote significant food restrictions to eliminate allergens or to cleanse the gastrointestinal system. These are all worthwhile endeavours, so the two-week phase of this diet should be seen as a positive thing and an attainable goal. Make no mistake, though, you will (and should) feel cravings and hunger pangs, and may go through some uncomfortable withdrawal symptoms. These are reminders of the comfortable sufficiency in which we normally live. It makes us mindful of the important reasons we have chosen to experience this hunger. Rest assured that no harm will come to you from feeling hungry during short periods of caloric restriction. Instead, allow these feelings to strengthen your resolve!

In this phase, sugar (white, brown, syrup, or honey); flour (baked goods of any kind—bread, buns, bagels, cakes, and cookies); pasta; rice; potatoes; soft drinks; fruit juices; and even fruits are eliminated. Obviously, when so many foods that may be dietary staples for a lot of people, are no longer consumed, you need to start eating alternatives such as salads, beans, nuts, whole grains, vegetables, fish, and lean meats (if you wish) as well as drinking more water.

In addition, it is important to eat your calories—not drink them. All caloric beverages need to be avoided, not just soft drinks and fruit juices, but milk shakes, fruit smoothies, milk, soy milk, as well as beer and wine or other alcoholic drinks. Only water, clear tea, and black coffee (no cream and sugar!) are permitted.

**PHASE TWO:** After two weeks, some initial weight loss has occurred—mainly through caloric restriction. At this point, whole fruits—but not fruit juices—are reintroduced, but baked goods, including all the "white foods" (sugar, flour, rice, pasta, mashed potatoes, and salt), are still eliminated in favour of whole unprocessed foods. Don't be misled by "whole grain" breads, pasta, or pizzas. Most of these do not contain intact grains; dough is made of processed grains which are milled into flour. There are some types of dark, heavy, chewy bread that have intact grains or sprouted grains. These can be introduced. Brown rice is permissible—white rice is not. Alcoholic beverages and all caloric drinks still need to be avoided.

This phase requires a lot of strength of will and determination, as well as resourcefulness in coming up with allowable meal choices. Phase Two continues for a minimum of four weeks or until the desired weight has been achieved. This is usually based on Body Mass Index and abdominal circumference measurement.

**PHASE THREE:** This is the long-term maintenance diet. It is essentially a reasonable diet based on whole, unprocessed foods, lots of grains, nuts, fruits, vegetables, fish, some low-fat dairy products, and lean meats if desired. Typically, you start with a good breakfast consisting of oats and other grains, or an egg, then a hearty lunch, a light dinner, and no after-dinner snacks. Make a point of consuming no calories after seven PM. You may feel hungry, yet no harm will come to you. Have some water or tea, and if you like, have some celery sticks or similar snack that is high in fibre and low in calories. Get used to light nutritious meals and avoid overeating. No particular food is disallowed, but dieters for the most part are wise to stick to the principles they learned in Phase Two. If weight is gained again, go back to Phase One.

The other guideline is to eat at least twenty different types of food each week, and rotate them, selecting at least ten new foods for the following week. This allows one to eat a large variety of different foods—grains, legumes, fruits, nuts, salads, veggies, fish, whole grain breads, et cetera, preferably when they are in season. Consuming a wide range of foods results in a greater exposure to important micronutrients. Not eating the same foods over and over again also reduces the likelihood of absorbing allergens and toxins.

Having a diversified diet (much like a diversified investment portfolio) gives us better exposure to a large variety of nutrients, in particular trace minerals and the thousands of phytochemicals that work synergistically and whose full effect on health and nutrition is not completely understood.

Try to follow the 90/10 Rule in any diet: if you stick to the optimal food choices 90 percent of the time, it is quite permissible to deviate 10 percent of the time.

Also—as with any other diet—a vigorous exercise program is an essential component to improve health and fitness. Diet alone is never enough.

........................................................................

*Why not?* thought David, as he left the good doctor's office. He knew he would not starve to death in two weeks if he stopped eating his morning croissant and orange juice. In fact, he could substitute hot oatmeal with ground flax and cinnamon for breakfast. Instead of his latte, he would forgo the whole milk and change to black coffee or green tea. He felt he had nothing to lose (except his twenty pounds!) and looked forward to being quicker on his feet again.

David remembered the "Flax Snax" that Jessica used to make for him when he went water skiing with some friends. They were little nuggets of goodness made with love that refuelled the men after a few rounds of slalom skiing. In fact, David's water ski coach used to quip that he did not particularly like skiing with David, but invited him along in the hope that he would bring some of his wife's tasty and nutritious treats. David thought he was just joking, but he could not be sure.

He felt that if he was going to be restricting calories now, he would need some nutrient-dense foods to keep his energy up. He emailed Jessica who was surprised by the request but happy to comply.

## FLAX SNAX

1 cup brown sugar
⅔ cup peanut butter or almond butter
½ cup maple syrup
½ cup melted butter
2 tsp. vanilla extract
3 cups quick-cooking oats
1 cup coarsely ground flax seeds
½ cup shredded coconut
½ cup sunflower seeds
½ cup raisins or dried cranberries
¼ cup wheat germ
6 Tbsp. sesame seeds
¼ cup pumpkin seeds

Heat oven to 350 degrees. Grease a 13 x 9 inch pan. In a large bowl, combine brown sugar, peanut butter, maple syrup, melted butter, and vanilla. Blend well. Stir in remaining ingredients. Press mixture evenly in prepared pan and bake for 15 to 20 minutes or until lightly brown. Cool completely. Cut into squares.

..........................................................................

Osler had stressed that any good diet program must be coupled with an exercise program, and David cycled over to the Peninsula Club for a core class; he took quiet pride in the fact that he was now regularly attending a variety of fitness sessions. That morning, he'd read a short section in *12 Habits* on the importance of core strengthening.

"Not that many years ago, men used to work out by bench-pressing and doing biceps curls. This would result in big chest and arm muscles but not necessarily good overall strength. Now the focus is largely on "core" conditioning, which strengthens the stabilizing muscles in the abdomen and back and improves balance and strength for most sports, as well as the activities of daily living. Think of the core as a "corset" or girdle, which gives strength and support to the entire trunk. This includes mainly the transverse and oblique abdominal muscles which also support the pelvis. It is important to work with a trainer to get a personalized and balanced fitness program, but a great way to strengthen the core muscles at home is to simply sit on an exercise ball while watching TV, or working at the computer.

After the exhausting class, David talked to one of the trainers who advocated taking a cold shower at the end of class. When he ran into Mary Ann at the water fountain, he mentioned this idea. She laughed. "I also practise 'hypothermic cardioversion.' That is, a cold shower will jump-start my heart."

"If I feel like I'm overheated after a workout, I'll often just have a cold shower to cool down." she continued. But if I'm not too hot after exercising, I'll take a steam bath to relax me and make me sweat, then have my cold shower. I find that most invigorating—the hot, then cold sensation revives me—and it also exercises the pores in my skin; the sweating and the heat open and cleanse the pores, and the cold closes them again."

While Mary Ann was enjoying a fruit smoothie, David opted for a pot of sencha green tea—mindful of his decision to avoid caloric drinks. She pulled out a bag of large cookies from her purse. "Have a Power Puck." she offered. "I was making some healthy home-made cookies for Erika's hockey team, and she asked me to make them without flour because one of her teammates was allergic to wheat. These are high in complex carbohydrates and protein, so they are great to refuel after a work-out or game." David was impressed, but as he was still in Phase One of the Osler Diet, he declined. However, he asked Mary Ann if she would share the recipe with him so he could make them later—and perhaps even impress Jessica and the kids!

**POWER PUCKS**

¼ cup butter
½ cup of chia gel
1 cup packed brown sugar
1 cup peanut butter
1 tsp. vanilla
3 free range eggs
3 cups old fashioned rolled oats
½ cup ground flax seeds
½ cup pumpkin seeds
½ cup dates
½ cup raisins
2 tsp. baking soda
Optional: 3-4 Tbsp. protein powder
1 cup semisweet chocolate chips

Preheat oven to 350 degrees. Lightly grease cookie sheets. Prepare chia gel by soaking two tablespoons of chia seeds in one cup of filtered water and let stand for ten minutes. Blend butter, sugar, peanut butter, and eggs in food processor or large bowl. Mix in baking soda, vanilla, oats, flax, pumpkin seeds, raisins, dates, and chia mixture until well blended. Scoop out dough by tablespoon. Press each cookie to flatten slightly. Bake fifteen minutes or until firm. Remove to wire racks to cool.

"Since I began eating more whole foods, and in particular whole grains, I've had fewer sugar cravings and better colonic evacuation," volunteered Mary Ann.

David was somewhat taken aback by his friend's candid description of her bowel activities until he remembered that Mary Ann, as a nurse, would have a pragmatic viewpoint about bodily functions.

"For breakfast, I will sometimes make hot oats, or muesli, or even toast made using a nice whole grain bread spread with nut butters, homemade preserves and cottage cheese." she continued. In each case, I then generously sprinkle my breakfast choice with what I call the "Holy Trinity of Seeds": chia, ground flax, and hemp hearts. When you buy the flax seeds, look for ones that are organically grown, grind them in a coffee mill, and store them in a glass jar in the refrigerator."

"Thank you, Mary Ann. Good advice," said David. "Do you have time to go for a short walk by the water?"

David realized he knew little about her life, apart from the fact she was a single mum and a nurse. "What has given you the most the most joy in your life?" he asked curiously.

Mary Ann smiled. "No surprise there, David. The safe

arrival of my children meant everything to me," she replied. "I thought I had it all in those early years. I was married to a surgeon who shared my interests in medicine, and who gave me financial security and the opportunity to live in a wonderful community. I was busy with Christopher and Erika, and although we did have some great moments as a family, I did not realize that Juan's career took precedence over everything else for him. Unfortunately, we did not survive as a couple. And when he had an affair with a recently-divorced colleague, I realized he had crossed the line. We separated and later ended the marriage. A bittersweet response to your question!"

"And yourself—what makes David tick?" she asked with a smile.

"Well, I've always been passionate about my work, but now, more than ever, I certainly agree that there is no greater joy than the birth of a child. This period of living away from my family while my wife and I try to sort things out has been lonely. The time for reflection has given me a tremendous opportunity to evaluate what is most important to me—and I now know that it is my family," responded David.

"I value our friendship a lot, Mary Ann. You have opened my eyes in many ways, and I hope we can build on that and stay in touch. But I need you to know that I'm resolved to go back to Jessica—if she'll take me."

Mary Ann nodded. "I thought that might be where you were headed, David. You're a changed man from the lawyer-in-a-hurry who was brought in on a stretcher to St. Luke's not so long ago."

On that note, they parted company but agreed to attend a stretching class together the following day and maybe chat afterwards.

# CHAPTER 12

*To change and to improve are two different things.*

**German proverb**

At his apartment, David brewed himself a clear chai tea. He had thought about making a chai latte with soy milk but remembered his plan not to drink any calories for two weeks. He sat upright on his exercise ball to engage his core muscles, and took out *12 Habits*.

As he was reading about the challenges of making positive and, he hoped, permanent lifestyle changes, it occurred to him that there were numerous parallels with his work in business law. A significant part of his practice involved working with organizations going through mergers, acquisitions, and other transitions. Many organizations seem to be in a constant state of change. Sometimes, in particular when someone new is at the helm, it may seem that there are changes, just for the sake of change. It is important to ensure that the change will be an improvement. People also change a lot: they grow, develop, evolve, react, age, get ill, and get better—or not. There is always the need to adjust to the new reality. As organizations change, the people in them must change as well; they must adapt or be left behind. David realized that the changes he was making were every bit as important as the ones he was managing for his clients—in fact more so. Were he not up to the task of living his life in a new way, he might not be able to return to the pressures of his work—and he had a family to support.

Since his heart attack, he certainly had a newfound sense of urgency. He understood the importance and relevance of eating well, taking the time to exercise, and getting sufficient sleep. More broadly, through meeting new friends such as Sanjay and Mary Ann, he'd become more aware of the purpose of his life. He also knew that he had to enter into a far more considerate relationship with Jessica and their children. David had a good support system: a healthcare team assembled through his cardiac rehab program, a sound working relationship with his family doctor, and staff at the Peninsula Club that motivated him.

David realized it was critical to have a clear vision of where he was going and he now had the desire to get there. He would build on what Sanjay had taught him: articulate the goal, create a detailed strategy of how to achieve it, and proceed confidently.

He knew he needed to take it a step at a time and that is exactly what he did. David was starting to enjoy cooking healthy meals for himself, his friends, and his family, and it was getting easier to do his workouts. In court, David had been known for his relentless pursuit of evidence that supported his position. He had no doubt that he could harness that determination now. Change is an emotionally-charged process. There is always fear and anxiety. Sometimes there is disillusionment—but if the change is positive and the purpose meaningful, there is also satisfaction and happiness. David perceived that by balancing all of the important aspects of his life, he would be able to make the changes stick.[84]

At David's follow-up medical appointment, Dr. Osler advised him that by his early forties, he needed to be proactive about his health above and beyond his heart disease risk. "In developed countries heart disease and stroke remain the most common cause of death, but cancer is a close second. Lung cancer is still the most lethal cancer, but among non-smoking men,

---

[84] Kotter, John. Principles of organizational change can be used as a metaphor for personal change. For a detailed discussion on organizational change management, see www.kotterinternational.com

prostate cancer and colorectal cancer are the most prevalent."

David intended never to smoke again, but at age forty-two he had given little thought to cancer screening. "I recommend that in addition to other blood work, you should consider having a PSA test done and a digital rectal exam," said Osler. "By the time you are fifty, you will also need a screening colonoscopy or at least an annual test for blood in the stool."

As David walked briskly back to his apartment, he reflected on his status as a middle-aged man, still young in many ways, but at the point where he must plan for the second half of his life, both in a physical and spiritual sense. Settling back with a cup of peppermint tea, he reached for *12 Habits*, and was once again amazed by the synchronicity of the book's ideas and his own thoughts.

*When we are no longer able to change a situation—just think of an incurable disease such as inoperable cancer—we are challenged to change ourselves.*

**Viktor Frankl** (1905–1997) Austrian neurologist and psychiatrist, Holocaust survivor, author of Man's Search for Meaning, published in German in 1946 and in English in 1963.

"

**HABIT ELEVEN: SEARCH FOR MEANING**

It turns out that the most important predictors of a good outcome following a heart attack are happiness in your marriage and job satisfaction. If someone is in a mutually-satisfying, loving relationship and also passionate about his work, this is better than any medication and more predictive of survival than family history, smoking history, blood pressure, or cholesterol level.

If you have ever witnessed the total personality change that can take place when someone falls in love and stays in love, you will agree that this joy is more valuable than gold. If this could be bottled it would be the most powerful and effective medicine there is.

.....................................................................

To develop a sense of purpose, activities such as doing interesting work (paid or volunteer), pursuing hobbies, and engaging in an active social life can help you set your compass. Try challenging yourself with music or language lessons, plan a trip with friends, or just hunker down with a good crossword puzzle on a weekend. And while you're at it, do it all with a smile. Studies show that a positive emotional state is also good for your brain. Happiness quotients have been measured; not only does spending time with happy people make you happier, but this effect continues to spread. So a smile can brighten someone's day, and they in turn are happier to the people they meet, and so on and so forth. In addition, not only do we smile when we *are* happy, but by smiling we can *become* happy. Conversely, by wearing a frown, we can make ourselves feel sad. It is fascinating that facial expressions influence our emotions, not solely the other way around.[85]

---

[85] Gladwell, Malcolm, *The Tipping Point*, 2000, chapter Two, (pages 78, and 84–87) discusses emotions going "outside-in," and in *blink*, 2005, chapter Six, (pages 197–208) he describes facial expressions as "action units." By practicing action units associated with various emotions, researchers actually experienced the emotion (for example, frowning would make one feel sad).

In living our lives with *meaning* we need to reflect on three important questions: What is my *purpose*? (Why am I here—at this place and in this time?) What is my *mission*? (What am I here to accomplish?) What is my *vision*? (What would I like the future to hold?)[86]

Where our *talent* (What am I good at?) and *passion* (What do I love to do?) intersect with what the world needs is our *calling*—the purpose of *life*.[87]

When life has meaning and one is successful, it becomes one's responsibility to share the lessons learned and help others to succeed as well. This is also the classic philosophy in medicine: "See one, do one, teach one." It is a way to spread the knowledge, but it is also a way to give back—to share one's blessings without any expectation of repayment. (Recall the section on volunteerism in Habit Five—Social Connection). *Leadership, then, is the obligation of people who are successful in their fields or have learned an important lesson that needs to be shared.*

*"With great power comes great responsibility."*

This was the lesson Spiderman learned in the comic books and movies. The quote is also found in speeches by American presidents—notably Franklin D. Roosevelt. But the original version of this credo can be attributed to Jesus Christ "From everyone who has been given much,

---

[86] Phillips, David, 2006, *Three Big Questions—everyone asks sooner or later, Canada*

[87] Wong, Davidicus, 21 March, 2009. PowerPoint presentation: *Surviving and Thriving as a Family Physician—What Quality Improvement means to me*. Burnaby, BC, Canada

much will be required; and from the one who has been entrusted with much, much more will be asked."[88]

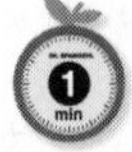

**One minute message**

In order to be *successful* and *happy*, there must be a good *reason* behind our actions. A life filled with *purpose* and *meaning* will be rewarding and satisfying.

Take the time to articulate the *objective* of your life—and what it is you wish to accomplish.

At the Peninsula Club after class, David invited Mary Ann to the juice bar to chat. "You've been a great friend to me through this ordeal," he told her. "You've helped me to realize so much about the spiritual dimension to recovery."

Mary Ann smiled. "I enjoy your friendship too, David. There aren't many men I've met who have been as willing as you to re-examine their lives."

"My heart attack was, in a way, a blessing for me," replied David. "The lessons I learned about eating better and exercising—as well as my appreciation for music and living in the moment—would not have happened if I'd not had a near brush with death. Someday I hope to be able to tell others about my experience so they won't have to go through a major health crisis in order to change their lifestyles."

"And I want you to know that you're a great role model, Mary Ann," David said with a smile. "Not only do you see

[88] Luke 12:48

the big picture, but you're trim and keep yourself in great shape. Is that a genetic disposition?"

"Not at all, David," said Mary Ann, acknowledging the backhanded compliment. "In fact I have a huge weakness for baked goods—croissants, fresh Italian bread, and pie are the top three. As my marriage was going on the rocks, I used food as an emotional outlet. Sure, I tried to lose weight, but diets didn't work for me. It was only when I realized that weight loss programs couldn't solve my problems that I began to gain control; I had to take matters into my own hands—and with that, my self-reliance gradually began to return."

"Rather than rewarding myself with a piece of warm chocolate fudge brownie and rich vanilla ice cream when I had a stressful day, I made an appointment for a Thai massage when I went a week without snacks and comfort foods." Suddenly, my weight was not the goal; it was about me now. As I continued to just eat well—a good breakfast, stop for a healthy lunch, then a light nutritious dinner, and no evening snacks—and take the time to walk every evening, the weight began to drop. It was not just the weight loss that made me feel happy again; it was realizing that I didn't need to take on all the problems of other people. I found that tremendously liberating."

"Ironically, I became successful in my weight loss only when I let go of my goal. Typically, we focus on objective outcomes when we describe success: how much money we make, how big a house we live in, how much we weigh, what car we drive, job promotions, conquests, and so on. It is important to set goals and take steps to achieve them, but I learned that by enjoying the journey I am more likely to reach my destination," said Mary Ann, sharing her wisdom.

*Success is peace of mind which is a direct result of self-satisfaction in knowing you did your best to become the best you are capable of becoming.*

Coach John Wooden (1910 – 2010)

From: *Pyramid of Success: Building Blocks for a Better Life*, John Wooden and Jay Carty.

Coach Wooden was the most successful college basketball coach, winning ten NCAA championships in twelve years with UCLA. However, he did not focus on winning, as he felt that was a by-product of preparation. Rather, he told his players, he was more interested in the process of becoming the best team they were capable of becoming.

The following week, Mary Ann joined David for a long bike ride. During a lunch break, he noticed that his usually bubbly friend was much quieter than usual. "What's up, Mary Ann?" he asked.

"Long story, David. It's about my sister."

"Tell me. I don't know anything about your siblings," said David.

"Lanai, who is three years younger than me, is in the Palliative Care Unit at St. Luke's with advanced cancer. She's the mother of four, has a career, is busy beyond belief, and didn't get around to having an abnormal pap smear repeated."

"Eventually, she had to have a physical for a life insurance policy, and when the pap smear results came back, she was referred for further testing. The diagnosis was invasive cervical cancer."

"She had a consultation at the cancer clinic with three gynecological cancer specialists: a gynecologic surgeon, a radiation oncologist, and a medical oncologist who prescribes chemotherapy. The consensus was that her best option would be a course of localized radiation as well as chemotherapy to shrink the tumour, and then surgery to remove it. Although there are no guarantees with cancer, the oncologists were confident that this intensive approach would be curative, as her disease had not metastasized."

"Lanai chose another treatment path," continued Mary Ann. "I was worried, but I know there is a fine line between assertively imposing one's values and beliefs on others versus letting adults make their own decisions."

"Fearing the toxicity of the proposed treatment, Lanai talked to friends and colleagues and researched alternative cancer treatment centres on the Internet. She decided on the Alpen Poliklinik, in Switzerland, which had successfully treated world leaders, entertainers, and business executives. She was very impressed by the clean and modern clinic in Geneva, as well as the friendly, professional staff. The doctor skillfully advanced a small catheter to the arteries supplying the tumour and then injected chemotherapeutic medications directly into the cancer. Lanai was told that this procedure increases the effectiveness and reduces the toxic side effects compared to injecting the drugs into a central catheter where they travel through the whole body. After two treatments the main tumour had shrunk modestly, but the cancer had invaded her intestine and had spread to her liver. As her bowel became obstructed, she needed to have a bowel resection done and came out of the OR with a colostomy. When she stabilized after the surgery she returned home but was booked to go back to Geneva in two weeks for more therapy."

"When Lanai arrived back in Canada, she was in unbearable pain and had dropped down to 90 pounds, having lost about a quarter of her body weight. She was seen in the ER at St. Luke's, given IV fluids, and her pain was treated. She began feeling a lot better a few hours after starting on narcotic medications, but even two days later she was still having so much abdominal pain that the staples from her surgical wound could not be removed. A CT scan confirmed that Lanai had significant spread of her disease to her liver as well as throughout her pelvis and abdomen."

"Their attending physician sat down with the family and told Lanai as frankly and gently as he could what the situation was. Dr. King went over the findings from the diagnostic studies done in Switzerland as well as Canada. He indicated that as the disease was no longer localized; it did not make sense to treat it only with localized chemotherapy. He also stated that Lanai was not alone in her desire to pursue alternative therapeutic options. 'Nobody seeks out an herbalist or chiropractor when they have acute appendicitis,' stated Dr. King. 'Clearly a skilled surgeon is needed. Some other diseases are not as straightforward, however, and cancer is certainly one of them. The treatment of localized disease by surgical resection is often curative if there has been no spread. However, if the cancer has metastasized, all bets are off, and nobody can guarantee a cure.'"

"Dr. King tried to deliver his message clearly and honestly while being careful to avoid blaming the patient for her condition or the choices she made. One can never know what the outcome may have been had a different treatment path been chosen. At the same time, he was careful to remain cautiously optimistic, while pointing out the futility of pursuing more treatments that were ineffective."[89]

"Paradoxically, many people who decline conventional therapy are brighter and more affluent than the average person. Of course, most individuals would not be able to afford medical treatments at a private Swiss clinic and so would simply accept the local options. Furthermore, these people have done a lot of research on the subject, and did not just accept the first solution they were offered. The research, however, is often done from their own lay perspective and comes from unsubstantiated or biased sources. The more one reads, the more one tends to 'overthink' the situation and the harder it becomes to make a decision or to accept the conventional approach. So it was with Lanai."

"My sister returned to the oncologist once again, this time willing to accept whatever advice had a reasonable chance of slowing down the progression of her cancer. Despite her weakened status and the extensiveness of the disease she had a fair chance of responding to standard therapy. She was considered to be relatively treatment naïve; that is, her tumour cells had not been exposed to a lot of chemotherapy and as such would be vulnerable to its therapeutic effect."

"The oncologist's position was that patients who choose alternative and unproven therapies should do so only when conventional treatments have failed. It is not unreasonable

---

[89] Posen, Dr. David B., 1994, *Always Change a Losing Game and Work-Life Balance*, Print and Tape editions. Albert Einstein stated that the definition of "insanity" was doing the same thing over and over again and expecting a different result. Dr. David Posen, an Ontario physician wrote an excellent self-help book entitled *Always Change a Losing Game*. In it he uses this sports metaphor to help the reader to identify and overcome harmful lifestyle habits.

for young patients in particular to 'go for broke' when treatments that have the highest chance of cure have been unsuccessful, but this should be done in the same way as patients are offered enrollment in clinical trials of new or unproven therapies—that is with informed consent as to the potential effectiveness and side effects. She emphasized that the most serious 'side effect' of choosing a harmless natural therapy is that it may delay the treatment of the cancer while it is still contained and curable."

"The oncologist also mentioned that there is a clinic in Vancouver that works in concert with the British Columbia Cancer Agency and provides integrated cancer treatment. They work both with patients who choose or decline conventional therapy. In each case the patient is instructed in healthy dietary and lifestyle choices and offered supplements that support the body's ability to fight cancer cells. The multidisciplinary team inspires patients to use whatever treatments resonate with their own values and beliefs. Conventional cancer therapy involves cutting out the cancer when possible or treating it with radiation beams or poisoning it with chemotherapy. None of these approaches support what the body does daily in locating and eliminating cancerous and precancerous cells. Recall that our immune systems destroy invading pathogens (viruses, bacteria, etc.) as well as cancerous cells. Regardless of what option a patient a chooses, the important thing is that they are informed of the chances of success and failure, and are aware of possible side effects as well as the consequences of not choosing therapy. At some point, patients may choose to decline therapy that they feel will adversely affect their quality of life without significantly extending their lives. As long as they reach this decision fully informed of all reasonable options, that is their right and as such needs to be respected by their family and care givers."

Mary Ann took a deep breath. "I asked Lanai if I could help her and her children prepare for the future. With the assistance of our family lawyer, I had all the appropriate papers drawn up and duly witnessed that would make me the executor of Lanai's estate and have power of attorney of a trust fund that would benefit her children. This done, Lanai and I were both filled with a sense of peace, knowing that no matter what happened to Lanai, her kids would be well looked after. These decisions have also freed my dear sister to concentrate on the task of healing," concluded Mary Ann. "Thank you for listening, David. You are a good friend."

# CHAPTER 13

*Life is like riding a bicycle. To keep your balance you must keep moving.*

**Albert Einstein**

Sanjay had given David a book that described numerous yoga poses, as well as the function of muscles and joints and how each may be beneficial. It also discussed the importance of breathing and included a detailed anatomic description of the structures required for respiration. Looking at an illustration of a single cell with its semi-permeable membrane, it occurred to David that the cell served as an analogy for balance within the body and more broadly for life itself. He learned that all living things must balance containment and permeability, rigidity and plasticity, persistence and adaptability, space and boundaries.[90]

*So be sure when you step. Step with care and great tact*
*and remember that Life's a Great Balancing Act.*
*And will you succeed? Yes! You will, indeed!*
*(98 and ¾ percent guaranteed)*

Dr. Seuss

"Oh the Places You'll Go!", 1990 —Theodor Seuss Geisel (1904–1991) American writer and cartoonist widely known for his children's books written under the pen name Dr. Seuss.

**HABIT TWELVE: A HEALTHY BALANCE**

Human beings are by far the most complex organisms on the planet. There is so much biological diversity and individual variation that it is impossible to give detailed recommendations on what constitutes a universally

[90] Kaminoff, Leslie, 2007, *Yoga Anatomy*, Human Kinetics, page 1

optimal diet and lifestyle. One size does not fit all. While there is consistency in the advice on what foods are healthy and what foods are not, certain individuals may not tolerate healthy foods because of specific medical conditions or allergies. Cost and availability are challenges as well. As much as possible, it is important to eat a wide variety of healthy foods to benefit from the richness and diversity of an optimal diet and reduce the risk of nutritional gaps due to overexposure to the same few ingredients.

It is abundantly clear that our bodies are designed to be active, and within reason, the more we move, the better. We all require aerobic fitness for endurance (to promote good cardiac and circulatory health) as well as anaerobic strength and conditioning training, along with flexibility and balance exercises to live fit and vital lives, prevent falls and fractures, and optimize function. There are dozens of benefits to exercise as detailed in Habit 2; however, you should be aware that over exercising can suppress immune function and lead to injuries or arthritis requiring joint replacements down the road. So again, the amount of exercise needs to be balanced and titrated to each individual.

It is also important to enjoy an occasional dessert or indulge in a glass of wine, without feeling that you are sabotaging your healthy lifestyle. As detailed earlier, smoking, drinking too much alcohol or coffee, using illicit drugs, and eating junk foods are harmful to our bodies. Yet, do not let a relentless pursuit of healthy living deny you the pleasures of sharing a piece of rich chocolate cake with family and friends on your birthday!

In addition to diet and exercise, there is good evidence to support the vital importance of social and spiritual connections, volunteerism, getting enough sleep, meditation, having passions, exploring the arts, and learning new skills. All of these pursuits improve our health and happiness; reduce the incidence of illnesses such as heart disease, cancer, dementia, and improve our chances of recovery or stability if we do get these conditions. But how much do each of us need? And how do we fit all these good things into our lives each day when we need to work and are busy with our families? How do we live our lives with purpose and meaning when we have to put food on the table, make the mortgage or rent payments, and ensure the kids get their homework done and make it to soccer and basketball practice on time? This is the challenge that all of us face to some degree, and this is why it is so critical to cultivate the Habit of Balance.

David had scheduled an appointment with Dr. Osler to bring him up to date on how he was doing. David had noticed that Osler's assistant, Sally, was a whirlwind of well-organized activity in the office. He remembered that at his law firm, he would usually give his urgent work to the busiest paralegal. *Is this because people who can create order out of chaos also know how to balance their activities and priorities?* he wondered.

"My heart attack has had a silver lining in that for the first time I am living my life with purpose and meaning," began David. "I am conscious that simple choices I make every day in terms of the foods I choose, the ways in which I exercise, or the time I take to see the beauty of nature, have made a tremendous difference to me. Now that I'm almost at the point of returning to work, I'm wondering if I can maintain these positive changes."

"As a physician, how do you manage to find balance in

your own life?" asked David.

"Well, physician health—including mental health and resilience—is often overlooked or taken for granted," replied Osler. "Historically, physicians were expected to work brutally long hours, and of course they could not 'call in sick'. So many physicians do not lead healthy lives and face burn-out. There is excellent work being done in the area of physician health and wellness now, but it was not even on the radar at all when I attended medical school."

"I remember a classmate who was struggling with depression and eventually dropped out. He was regarded as weak by his classmates and somehow unfit to become a doctor. Since I started my practice I've known a few colleagues who had mental health or substance misuse issues. One was an anesthesiologist with a narcotic addiction. Over the years he became an expert in hiding it. He avoided injecting in the bathroom so he did not have to hide needle marks, but inserted a Foley catheter into his rectum with the opening pinned to the inside of his scrub pants. It became easy when giving a patient fentanyl to save part of the dose and inject it into his catheter. The drug would simply get absorbed through the rectal mucosa. Eventually, he was discovered, as a medication audit showed that he was using more fentanyl than other anesthesiologists with a similar case load. He came clean and admitted his addiction. He was suspended and spent three months away from work receiving treatment at a residential rehab facility that specialized in treating doctors with dependency disorders."

Osler stated that—knock on wood—he had lived a charmed life.

"I could certainly do with more money and fewer days in the office, but I really can't complain. I try hard to take care of myself; Madeline and I enjoy making healthy meals taste great; and I love to go hiking and kayaking on weekends. Early on, I deliberately found a congenial group to work with, which enables me to take time off to spend with my family. I used to think it was a bit selfish, but now I realize that if I don't take care of myself I can't look after my patients either."

"I'm also aware that despite my best efforts, many factors are out of my control, and I have learned not to take my well-being for granted. I'm a big believer in proactive lifestyle interventions, as you know, but sometimes illnesses can hit you like an asteroid from outer space, and all you can do is react. When I hear about an unexpected illness or injury, a bereavement or separation, a financial catastrophe or other misfortune, I think, 'Man, that could be me; there but for the grace of God go I.'"

After the appointment, David cycled to False Creek, sat down on a quiet bench and pulled out *12 Habits*:

> " Cardiac surgeons used to believe that about 90 percent of the risk for heart disease was genetic. If that were true, choosing your parents carefully would be the most important undertaking when trying to control heart disease. Fortunately, this is incorrect, and as the landmark international (Canadian-led) "INTERHEART Study" pointed out, specific—mostly controllable—risk factors predict 90 percent of heart disease risk.
>
> Health researchers have recently discovered that regardless of where you live or whatever your age, gender, or race is, 90 percent of first heart attacks (myocardial infarction) can be attributed to nine risk factors. They include: cigarette smoking, an abnormal ratio of blood

lipids, high blood pressure, diabetes, abdominal obesity, stress, a lack of daily consumption of fruits and vegetables, as well as a lack of daily exercise. Modest alcohol consumption (three to four drinks weekly) has been determined to be a preventive measure.

INTERHEART is a global study led by McMaster University's Dr. Salim Yusuf that focuses on cardiovascular disease (CVD) and was co-funded by the Canadian Institutes of Health Research (CIHR), the Heart and Stroke Foundation of Ontario, and thirty-seven other funding sources. The study involved 15,000 patients with a first acute myocardial infarction (AMI) and 15,000 asymptomatic control subjects (age and sex matched) who were drawn from 262 centres in 52 countries throughout Asia, Europe, the Middle East, Africa, Australia, and North and South America.

Structured questionnaires were administered and physical examinations were undertaken in patients and in controls. Information was gathered about demographic factors, socioeconomic status, lifestyle, personal and family history of CVD, and psychosocial factors. Non-fasting blood samples were taken from every individual and frozen immediately after processing for later analysis. Waist measurements and hip circumferences were recorded.

Current smokers were defined as individuals who had smoked any tobacco in the previous twelve months and included those who had quit within the past year. Former smokers were defined as those who had quit more than a year earlier.

All of this information was sent to the Population Health Research Institute, McMaster University, and Hamilton

> Health Sciences for quality control and statistical checks. The effect of these nine risk factors is consistent in men and women, across different geographic regions, and by ethnic group, making the study applicable worldwide. Among implications of the study, the concept of a uniform, balanced, preventive strategy for heart attack across the world appears to have great potential impact. The ways in which the heart attacks that follow from the nine risk factors reflect the interplay of environmental and constitutional (genetic) influences remain to be further explored.[91]

David found this study intriguing and empowering. It seemed intuitive to him that the risk factors for heart disease were largely controllable. Here was empirical proof. As luck would have it, he was meeting Sanjay at the Teahouse in Stanley Park that afternoon to learn more about Magna Vita.

The two men decided to take a table outside and enjoy the view. David remembered to wear his sunglasses—and not just to look like a mysterious movie star. Dr. Osler had told him of the importance of UV light exposure in causing skin cancers, photoaging and wrinkles, as well as visual deterioration because of cataracts and macular degeneration.

"Think of sunglasses as sunscreen for your eyes," Osler had said. "Wear your sunglasses for driving and hiking, or if you require glasses to correct your vision, make sure to get a UV filter layer applied to them."

---

[91] Yusuf, Salim, et al., 2004, Effect of potentially modifiable risk factors associated with myocardial infarction in 52 countries (The INTERHEART Study): case-control study, *The Lancet*, vol. 364, no. 9438, September 11.

"Sanjay, do you have any tips on weight reduction? I need to trim about twenty pounds as part of my recovery," asked David, as he looked at the menu.

"Funny you should ask, as I've actually thought about this quite a lot," replied Sanjay. "As you know, being overweight is also a major risk factor for me. I have just compiled a simple fact sheet on the subject. Why don't you have a quick look?"

**What Determines Body Weight?**

**1. How Much you eat.** Clearly the more one eats, the more one weighs. To lose weight, the most important thing is to cut back the calories.

**2. How Fast you eat.** Faster eaters are more likely over-eaters and more likely to be obese than are those who eat slowly and mindfully. Think about your food and where it came from and how if got to your table. Savour your food while you reflect upon it in gratitude to those who grew your food, harvested it, transported it, prepared it, and served it to you.

**3. What you eat.** Consuming a diet high in refined carbohydrates only makes sense if you are very active and burn those calories. Otherwise they go into storage as fat. So focus on whole, unprocessed foods.

**4. When you eat.** People often skip breakfast, eat a quick lunch, then have a big dinner when they get home and snacks in front of the TV to relax in the evening. Calories taken in at the end of the day have no chance of getting burned. It makes more sense to redistribute those calories earlier in the day when we are more active. Challenge yourself to stop consuming any calories after seven PM—it won't kill you.

**5. Who you are.** The rate at which each individual metabolizes energy is based on that person's exercise level, body composition, and genetic predisposition.

> Try the Raisin Meditation. Take a raisin and sit down comfortably. Pick it up and think about where it was grown. Think of the sun drenching the vineyard in California and how long the vines have been there, who planted them and tended them. Reflect on the vine through the growing season, buds, tiny green grapes, then after months of sun and rain, plump ripe dark purple grapes. These are harvested and laid in the sun to dry. Then they are packed and shipped to where they are purchased. Look at the raisin carefully and smell it. Anticipate the sweet and succulent taste. Savour it slowly, swallow and feel it go down and let it nourish you. When you have finished you will probably notice two things—it has never taken that long to eat a raisin, and it has never tasted better. Apply this mindful eating to your next meal.

David decided to forgo the bread basket and opted for his now familiar, somewhat austere, but delicious selection of organic greens with grilled salmon.

When I attended college in India," said Sanjay, "I competed in track and field. I was a decathlete, and enjoyed the challenge and variety of training for ten different, but related events. Learning how to live well is similar, in that it is wonderful to excel in any one discipline, but true satisfaction and meaning comes from balancing all *12 Habits*. That is why I founded the Magna Vita Institute."

David regarded him with some awe. It had just dawned upon him that Sanjay had not only founded the Institute but also written the book.

"I feel that we could all do with a makeover, David," continued Sanjay. "We live busy lives and too often rush from one appointment to another. We take on debt to buy expensive homes and cars, take lavish holidays to impress ourselves and our friends, and then become enslaved to long hours at work to support this lifestyle."

"Remember the old joke that nobody on their deathbed wishes they had spent more time at the office? But the truth is that not enough of us live our lives with purpose and meaning. Coaching ordinary people to improve their relationships and their health in the full sense of the word is the mission of the Magna Vita Institute. In this way, people can learn to live extraordinary, balanced, and happy lives."

"I'll tell you what I've learnt, Sanjay, from studying *12 Habits*. You were the first person after I left hospital to point me to the nutrition and lifestyle changes necessary to achieve good health. And the more I read your book, the more I realize there are common themes. The same changes that help me to reduce my risk of heart disease also reduce my risk of stroke, diabetes, Alzheimer's disease, cancer, arthritis, osteoporosis, and depression. That is impressive!"

"At the same time, practising the *12 Habits* improves the metabolism and immune system—helping one to achieve optimum weight, reducing allergies and infections, and improving alertness, energy, and sleep. In this manner, we can literally slow our own aging process. I don't just mean looking and feeling younger, although that's important. But we can also diminish the risk of the four age-related conditions that we fear the most: cardiovascular disease (heart disease and stroke); neurodegenerative disorders (such as Parkinson's disease and dementia); musculoskeletal degeneration (osteoarthritis and osteoporosis); and cancer."

"I see now that there are also similarities among diverse healing systems. Each one enjoys numerous healing successes, and yet, curiously, none seems to work for all illnesses. But I think there is a final common pathway for healing. I've been reading about the power of a "therapeutic encounter." By listening attentively to a person's story and validating their experience, and then giving them genuine support and compassion, this encounter can be a catalyst to begin a cascade of healing that can have powerful results. Most physicians have had the experience of a patient saying 'I feel ever so much better, just having talked to you, doctor.' All of that can occur even without specific medications or physical therapies, such as prescription pills or surgery or even supplements, needling, manipulation, or other forms of body work!"

The "Placebo Response" of noting improvement without active therapy is so well known that all drug trials need a placebo (or control) group to sort out what the true effect of the medication is. Yet the placebo response is often much greater that the effect of the active treatment. It would be safe and powerful medicine indeed if we could harness the healing power of the placebo response in a therapeutic encounter.

The meal was over, but David and Sanjay continued to talk late into the afternoon. David was clearly in an expansive mood. "Even as I look at different religions I feel that there are more similarities than differences. The teachings of the Buddha, Jesus the Christ, Muhammad, and the gurus all instruct followers to lead honest lives and be respectful of others. Christianity asks that you love and worship God, respect all of creation, and treat your neighbour as you would like to be treated. Buddhism teaches loving kindness and non-violence as a way of life. Both teachers, although separated by five hundred years, three thousand miles, and vastly different cultures and languages, used similar words to speak of compassion, forgiveness, and 'the way' or path to the 'one truth'.[92]

"You've obviously been doing a lot of thinking and reading, David. You've taken the time to reflect on the world around you," said Sanjay. "For my part, it makes little difference which belief system is practised, as many of them have the potential to address the spirituality, which connects us. In fact, I feel that it may be just as good for me to become more spiritual without following any specific religion. I agree with you that we should be tolerant of different faith groups. I also think the same should apply to different forms of healing."

"Let me tell you about a friend in Alberta. Liz Barker is a doctor who loves to ride horses. A few years ago, she fell and suffered a severe ankle fracture. It eventually healed, but she developed a painful complication called reflex sympathetic

---

[92] Borg, Marcus, 2002. Editor: *The Parallel sayings of Jesus and Buddha*, Duncan Baird Publishers, London.
As Buddha caused a renewal movement within Hinduism, so too did Jesus in Judaism; yet neither saw himself as a founder of a new religion.

dystrophy (RSD). This is a neurological condition marked by burning pain, sweating, swelling, as well as changes to the skin and muscles in the region. She sought the advice of numerous orthopedic specialists to get relief of her constant pain and cramping, which had resulted in a deformity of her left foot. Each specialist told her that there was little that could be done for this condition. No longer able to work, she attended a pain clinic and was given narcotics to take on a regular basis. This helped, but left her feeling mentally slow as well as constipated. She was advised that the only permanent solution would be an amputation below her knee and to get used to walking with a prosthesis."

"As you can imagine, Liz did not relish the thought of having her left lower leg amputated. Also, she could not be assured that she would not develop RSD in the stump. A friend told her of Dr. Stephanie Aung, a Chinese-trained doctor who practised Western medicine as well as Traditional Chinese Medicine (TCM). She had had some success treating pain conditions. Liz decided to pay her a visit and began experiencing relief through the use of acupuncture and other therapies."

"Incredibly, Liz improved to the point that she was able to return to work on a part-time basis. She visited the orthopedic surgeon who had recommended an amputation as her only option and told him of the success she had had through TCM. He responded by waving his hand dismissively. 'I am glad you are better, Liz, but I don't understand or believe in alternative medicine, and I don't think that's what helped you. In my opinion, you were just lucky.' Liz now has a new mission: she is determined to find ways to bridge the gulf between practitioners of western and alternative forms of healing."

*Out beyond ideas of wrongdoing and rightdoing, there is a field. I'll meet you there.*

**Rumi** (1207–1273) mystical Persian poet and Muslim philosopher.

As they parted company for the afternoon, Sanjay challenged David to use the 12 Habits to balance spirit, mind, and body and to keep him at the top of his game. "Being at our peak performance for work, play, and interpersonal interactions is just as important as a professional athlete staying in shape," said Sanjay. "Imagine if a player showed up for a game having slept poorly, being overweight, out of shape, jittery from coffee, and not mentally prepared. Why is it any different in our lives? In our work and our interactions with family and others we can choose to be alert, prepared, and mindful—or not."

"Remember that it's also necessary to develop the skills to internalize the habits. Just as an athlete or a musician needs to train or practise daily, it's not enough to follow a new way of living only once in a while; fundamental and consistent changes are required to optimize health outcomes."

**One minute message**

Throughout our lives, we are frequently faced with competing interests and options. We can *choose* to make a healthy meal, or grab some fast food. We can *choose* to get exercise, or to relax in front of the TV with a beer. We can make the *choice* to stop destructive behaviours and habits, or not. We can *choose* jobs and relationships that resonate with who we are, or settle for mediocrity.

This is the *Magna Vita Moment*: We can *choose* to follow the path of least resistance, or we can conscientiously live our lives with purpose and meaning. We can be role models of a healthy lifestyle and in doing so be a motivation and inspiration to others. At the same time, these choices will enrich our own lives and help us achieve optimal health, balance, and happiness.

One of David's primary goals was to re-establish his relationship with Jessica and return to the family. He had not been surprised to read that the happiness that stems from a loving relationship trumps the satisfaction that comes from one's job, community, or financial success. When Jessica agreed to join him on a hike in Manning Park one Sunday, he was elated. They parked near a trail head and walked for the first hour in a silent meditation, reverently taking in the beauty of the mountains and the fragrant alpine meadows. At a breathtaking viewpoint, David pulled a blanket out of his back pack and invited her to have a snack. He had brought cheese and whole-grain crackers, apples, frozen green grapes, and his own trail mix of nuts and seeds with some dried fruits and candied ginger. They washed this feast down with some refreshing water. "This is wonderful," said Jessica, smiling at David. "I didn't have to organize a thing!"

They chatted about Jessica's work, David's recovery, things that were good about their relationship and challenges that they still faced. They talked about their hopes and dreams for Adam and Rebecca. "Through my illness and recovery, I'm learning to be a bit more like you," said David.

"In what way, David?" she asked curiously.

"I realize that I am a bit of a perfectionist and can be demanding to a fault. I have always had very high expectations for myself and don't tolerate anything less of my colleagues and employees. I spent more time at the law office than I did at home, but I suspect that I maintained that attitude with you and the kids as well."

"It's no wonder Adam and Rebecca don't want me to help them with their homework and school projects. I've always told them that they would not succeed if they settle for mediocrity; but if the bar is raised too high, it makes the goal unattainable as well; 'perfect is the enemy of good.'"[93] You have always been more patient and felt that sometimes 'good enough' is okay. I realize that you are right, and I have decided to relax a bit more and try to let go. I'm not sure that I'm ready to wear my heart on my sleeve, but I need to be more open with my thoughts and feelings and fears. Maybe I can open my heart—physically and figuratively!"

They packed up and headed back to the car. When David dropped her off at the family home, it was Jessica who invited him in to have a cup of tea and to spend some time with the kids.

.........................................................................

As David prepared to return to the law office and the demands of his practice, he grew wary that the lessons of 12 Habits might go by the wayside. How was he going to

---

[93] Voltaire (1694–1778). *Le mieux est l'ennemi du bien.* Often, trying too hard or pushing too much will not result in the desired outcome as the cost is too great, and unintended adverse outcomes may result. We see this in medicine when we try too aggressively to reach targets for blood pressure or blood sugar control only to see the consequences of hypotension and hypoglycemia (dizziness, falls, fractures, confusion).

balance his competing interests? He called Sanjay to see if he had time for tea. The taxi driver had a couple of hours before he went on shift, so they arranged to meet at a café not far from David's apartment.

"I'm worried, Sanjay. Many times what we need to do—make a living—takes precedence over what we want to do—have a life. I'd love to work out for two hours a day, practice yoga and meditation daily, and take the time to prepare healthy, locally-sourced meals and share them in peace with my family and friends. I want to hike and travel more, learn languages and new instruments, and spend meaningful time with my wife, children, and close friends. But I also need to work—which I actually enjoy most days—and I need sleep! How am I going to be able to get it all in?"

Sanjay smiled. "A full and busy life is a blessing indeed. You are very fortunate that you have so many interests and opportunities. You're in the enviable position where you can choose from many good options. Sometimes we need to sacrifice some things that we cherish for a greater good. Parents often sacrifice their desperately-needed sleep to get up with their crying infants or sick children. It is one thing to give our time and money to our family and friends, but we may also feel compelled to give resources that we ourselves need to support charities or other deserving causes. So sacrifice involves giving up something good for something that we feel is even more important."

"When choosing among multiple, competing options in our daily lives, we need to decide whether it is worth sacrificing our time with the family, for example, for an opportunity at career advancement—which may involve more travel away from home. And that's true of leisure time too; it's great to play hockey with the boys and drop by the bar afterwards, or go away for a spa weekend with friends, but if it comes at the cost of precious time away from the family, we need to evaluate what's most important."

"Personally, I feel that when I can't pack everything into a day, I need to prioritize. I know I need to exercise regularly, but when I'm tired, *sleep trumps exercise*. In the same way, I need to earn a living, but when it comes down to it, *family trumps work*. And most times, healthy food choices win over tempting snacks. It's similar with social and career opportunities; we can't do it all. This obviously means saying 'No' to many things. I have come to realize, however, that saying 'No' to things that are less important allows me to say to say 'Yes' to things that are more in line with my personal mission, values, and beliefs."

**One minute message**

Learning to say *no* to certain things automatically means saying *yes* to others.

When our plates are *full*, agreeing to get involved in interesting opportunities requires us to make room by dropping other commitments and responsibilities. *Be careful* what you agree to take on, and ensure it is not at the expense of your important core values.

"I hear you, Sanjay. I need to work to pay my bills, and I need to sleep, so how do I make time for exercise or having fun?" asked David."

"You may not be able to get up early every morning and

exercise, but you can surely get up early once or twice a week to attend a gym class or yoga class," replied Sanjay. "Remember that some exercise is always better than none. It is not easy making the time for exercise, but like many things in life, making the effort is worthwhile. Exercise is also invigorating; it actually gives you more energy."

"Fitting everything in that you want to do is not easy; it requires planning and effort. Mediocre effort does not often lead to success. The truth is that hard work, determination, and even self-sacrifice are often required to reach our goals. I remember when I was in high school my mother gave me a plaque which read, 'Opportunity is often missed because it is disguised as hard work', Sanjay recalled with a smile."

"Reaching health goals—like quitting smoking, losing weight, or competing in a triathlon—or personal goals such as getting admitted to medical school or other professional college, receiving a promotion at work, or becoming financially independent are all hard work. In the same way, staying healthy and fighting the ravages of aging is *like swimming against the current*. The natural tendency *is not to succeed*. This is why we must refuse to give in to the path of least resistance."

"Salmon work hard to swim upstream to spawn and reproduce their species. It may seem like a powerful tide is washing us out to sea, but we need to put in a herculean effort to avoid getting tossed into the rocks where our broken carcasses will be eaten by the gulls and crayfish! Many times, hard work will be rewarded and we will reach our goals. Often, the greater the effort, the greater the reward—however, this is not always the case, because life is not fair. Yet, it is still important for our self-satisfaction to give our best in all we do. Doing the best we are capable of is a better marker of success than achieving a particular outcome."

**One minute message**

The path of least resistance rarely leads us to a desired destination. *Magna Vita* is possible; we may have to *work* for it, however.

We need to be willing to stubbornly *fight the tide* that is washing us out to sea in order to reach our personal goals and health objectives.

Sanjay had to admit that he often felt his life was like trying to walk on a log in the water. It's easy to fall off and struggle to get back on. He enjoyed practising hot yoga, but even that was a love-hate relationship. He hated getting up early to attend, he hated feeling lightheaded and nauseous in class, and he hated falling out of the poses awkwardly. However, he absolutely loved the way he felt after a class, and he was getting stronger, leaner, more flexible, and his *balance was improving*. In addition, by practising regularly, he felt that he had sharper concentration as well as more determination and patience in many aspects of his life. Furthermore, the breath work he had learned and "stillness at your edge" were skills that were transferrable to other aspects of his life.

"Sanjay, I couldn't agree with you more about the necessity for me to create a better work-life balance," said David. "But I wonder how it's possible to achieve in a law office.

"Many of us can flex our work schedules to some extent," replied Sanjay. "I'm not talking about deceitfully calling in sick on a regular basis because you feel you 'deserve' a day off. I'm talking about working with your partners and associates to either come in early some days and leave early or come in late some days. Try taking an earned day off every two weeks by doing an extra hour a day, or simply negotiating a less than full-time position. A 0.8 Full Time Equivalent (FTE) gives you one day off a week, and a 0.9 FTE gives you 90 percent of your salary and a half day off each week to catch up on whatever you want to do. The improvement in lifestyle and satisfaction usually more than compensates for the small reduction in pay. You are often happier and more productive in the work environment as well when you do not resent your employment for making you miss out on significant aspects of your life."

"Perhaps I can build this into my schedule when I return to work," said David thoughtfully. "I'll be starting on a graduated timetable anyway. If I slot exercise periods and important family events into my calendar, it won't fill up automatically with commitments not consistent with my own priorities. I'll go over my day planner tomorrow with my assistant and block off some of these essential gaps. A friend told me recently that if I don't make time for myself, I won't be there for clients or family either," said David, remembering Mary Ann's words.

"The other thing that you will undoubtedly notice," Sanjay said, "is that things tend to spiral in life. Do you remember our conversation about mind-body medicine and how belief affects healing? When some things in life are going well, you get on a roll, and other aspects are good too. But if you have a bad day at work, an upsetting relationship issue, a financial setback, whatever, it seems that everything spirals downwards.

You have to be aware of that and not let one negative event spoil your whole day—or year—or life. Look for the positives. Do meaningful work, spend time with optimistic people, eat well and stay healthy, let go of anger, forgive others, spend time connecting spiritually to a reality bigger than ourselves. And whatever you do, choose to do it with a smile—letting your joy and happiness radiate out to others.[94]

"When all of these habits are incorporated into our lives and reverberate in balance it is like a beautiful cord played on a twelve-string guitar ...twelve strings, different notes, but all resonating in one glorious harmonic sound!"

"And that brings me to the graduation ceremony, David," Sanjay said with a proud smile. "You have worked very hard since your heart attack, and have made changes in your life that have improved your health immensely—your health in the full sense of the word—physical, emotional, mental, spiritual, and communitarian. This has made you happier and more fulfilled than you have been in years and has also improved the key relationships in your personal life and community. I feel that you exemplify the vision of the Magna Vita Institute, and so it is my privilege to bestow upon you the Magna Vita Medallion."

With that, Sanjay presented David with a small jeweller's box. David opened it and took out a gold medal about the size of a half-ounce maple leaf gold coin with the letters "MV" embossed on one side. It was attached to a gold chain, which

---

[94] Bach, R., 1977. This principle is what Richard Bach called "Cosmic Law" in his book *Illusions, the Adventures of a Reluctant Messiah*: "Like attracts like. Just be who you are, clear and calm and bright. Automatically, as we shine who we are ... that turns away those who have nothing to learn from who we are and attracts those that do, and from whom we have to learn as well." ( pages 146–147)

David hung around his neck, tucking the medal into his shirt.

David looked at his friend and smiled in return. He was sitting here with this amazing, insightful man who had come from half way around the world to be his inspiration and his teacher. A few short months ago David had suffered a heart attack and could have died. Instead, he was reborn. Sanjay earned his living as a cab driver, and yet like so many people, when the surface is scratched, a marvelous and complex character is revealed. Why had it taken a heart attack for David to discover some simple truths about himself and his priorities? He could not answer that question, but he was immensely grateful that he had gained Magna Vita—a full and meaningful life.

David was filled with a sense of satisfaction as he walked back to his apartment. He felt he had the *obligation of the cured*. He wanted to share his new-found knowledge and wisdom. He felt responsible for becoming a catalyst for change rather than waiting for others to do something. He remembered reading the words of Mahatma Gandhi, "You must be the change you wish to see in the world."

David decided to indulge in his favourite hot beverage: a matcha soy chai latte. He mixed some matcha tea with hot water and used his bamboo whisk to beat it to a smooth frothy liquid. He brewed the spicy chai tea and steamed the soy milk. He blended it together and sprinkled some cinnamon on top. Then he sat down to enjoy the fine balance of antioxidants and exotic flavours, secure in the knowledge that something this tasty was also good for him. It was well worth the effort—and the calories. He had lost seven pounds already and rarely drank any calories as recommended in the Osler Diet, but this was one of those exceptions that he allowed himself under the "90/10 Rule."

David Mackenzie, a reinvented forty-two-year-old man, opened his book to the last page. He read the conclusion and nodded; he could not believe how far he had come in such a short period of time.

> "Our bodies are designed to be healthy and desire to be happy. We need to cultivate the appropriate habits that will allow us to optimize our health and avoid pitfalls that sabotage success. In doing so, we can reach our full potential and live a vibrant life of purpose, meaning, harmony, and balance.

David grasped the medallion around his neck. Like an Olympic athlete who could not quite believe he had won a gold medal, he stuck it in his mouth and bit it. It was real.

Maybe now an ordinary lawyer could indeed live an extraordinary life.

# EPILOGUE OR … WHY I WROTE THIS BOOK

*To cure sometimes, to relieve often, to comfort always—this is our work. This is the first and greatest commandment. And the second is like unto it: Thou shalt treat thy patient as thou wouldst thyself be treated.*

**Anonymous**: the first nine words are attributed to Hippocrates and to Dr. Edward Trudeau (1848–1915), founder of Adirondack Cottage Sanitarium, New York, in 1885.

I could have called this book, as my wise mother suggested, "What Every Patient Should Know." As a physician for over twenty years, I have noticed a significant number of recurring themes when I give advice to my patients. As I am not able to see nearly all of the people who have asked to come into the practice, this book gives me an opportunity to reach a wider audience. My hope in writing *One Minute Medicine* is that it will empower readers to improve their own health.

I chose the title *One Minute Medicine*, as I believe even one-minute interventions and one good idea can be life changing. In the blink of an eye, someone may decide to stop smoking, make small but meaningful dietary changes, and embrace a healthier lifestyle. Many people feel overwhelmed when facing a challenge—be it losing 50 pounds, getting fit, completing a marathon, learning a new language, quitting bad habits, or adjusting a work schedule to achieve balance in life. It is important to remember why we are making the change and how our lives will be better after having reached our goal. Nonetheless, it can be discouraging to have a big goal that is difficult to reach, and often we may have tried before—and failed.

We must remain determined and persistent as we keep the goal in mind, and visualize what success will look like—but we must also stay in the moment and focus on what we can do today—now—in the next minute. Like the Zen expression "The journey of a thousand miles must begin with a single step," my hope is that this book will serve as the motivation to enable readers to take that first important step. For many of us, it will not be the first time that we have come across this information, yet perhaps this book will provide a catalyst for meaningful change.

I should make it clear that One Minute Medicine in no way endorses the "hand on the door-knob" or "fast food" style of health care practised in many HMOs and walk-in clinics in North America today. I believe this is a poor way to deliver primary care, and in particular manage chronic disease.

At the heart of a family physician's expertise is the ability to *synthesize* vast amounts of information—often from disparate sources—and *communicate* it effectively, via longitudinal relationships spanning multiple family members and over many years. In addition, the family physician strives to provide his or her patients timely screening and early detection of major medical conditions, appropriate acute care, and chronic disease management, along with mental health treatment in order to preserve function and independence and thereby reduce hospitalizations and infirmity. Ideally, family physicians should also support their patients with lifestyle coaching and disease prevention leading to optimal health and happiness.

Many of the anecdotes and stories in these pages are drawn from my clinical practice and experiences. However, this is a work of fiction, and any names or specific examples that may resemble actual people or events are purely coincidental. Most are composites drawing on several cases that are pulled together to illustrate a particular point.

I should also state that I do not consider myself an expert in the fields of nutrition, fitness, cardiology, cancer care, relaxation and spirituality, or motivation. Many of these ideas in *One Minute Medicine* are not new, nor are they mine alone. Some of my favourite thinkers and mentors in the field of healthcare and "selfcare" are listed in the references. However, I believe that the generalist is in a unique position to look at health in a broad sense and give an overall and balanced perspective of factors which influence health and illness.

I wanted to join together the concepts and thoughts gleaned from the perspective of two decades of clinical practice into a concise and practical form that would be accessible to as many people as possible, some of whom are undoubtedly more versed than I in the topics discussed, and others for whom these ideas may be new. This bringing together of various habits and practices is part of the field of Integrative Medicine, a term coined by Dr. Andrew Weil. Integrative Medicine describes a healing-oriented system involving the spirit, mind, and body, which evaluates and embraces all therapies and interventions—both conventional and alternative. It is grounded in science and neither accepts nor rejects any practices blindly, but aims to incorporate less harmful practices when possible that stimulate the body's innate ability to heal itself. A priority is promotion of health and prevention of illness through education, as well as treatment of disease. In a tangible manner, our health is affected by our environment, so Integrative Medicine is also concerned with protection of our natural environment as well as the stressors that contaminate our personal environments.

As some of the concepts discussed in this book are peripheral to standard medical teaching, *One Minute Medicine* is my attempt to nudge some of these practices a little more into the mainstream. Clinicians should maintain a robust scepticism when it comes to examining unfamiliar practices and therapies. One can—and should—question therapies that seem too good to be true, while remaining open-minded to the possibility that they may indeed be true. Lack of evidence of benefit is not the same as evidence of lack of benefit; many traditional therapies may be safe and useful even if randomized controlled trials, the gold standard of medical evidence, have not been conducted. Conversely, the more toxic a therapy, the greater the burden of proof for effectiveness must be. For very serious illnesses, it is also important to bear in mind that a potentially fatal adverse reaction to a gentle natural therapy might be that its use results in the delay of effective conventional therapy at a time when it may still be curative.

I am also acutely aware of the importance of *physician health*; physicians are not always the best role models for a healthy lifestyle, and many have not achieved balance in their own lives. In some cases, this leads to tragic events resulting in a physician being lost to their patients, their family, and to society. Furthermore, evidence now supports what was always intuitively obvious: patients under the care of a physician who makes his or her own health and wellbeing a priority achieve better health outcomes than those who do not. So I hope that this book will be an asset to physicians as a tool that they can use in their own lives and practices.

More broadly, this principle applies to all of us who in some way or another provide care for people. If we, as physicians, parents, teachers, and others in caregiving or leadership roles, do not make the effort to look after ourselves, and work to achieve balance in our own lives, we will be of little use to those who depend on us. Along the way we will risk burn-out, unhappiness, poor health, and premature death.

While there is a greater complexity and sub-specialization in medicine than ever before, there is also a greater need for generalist physicians to make sense of the numerous facets of healthcare to avoid fragmentation of care. There is also a greater need for self-care. Although physicians need to be knowledgeable and skilled care providers and resources for patients, I believe that we are all responsible for looking after ourselves; we need to take a proactive role in being well and whole. My brother, for example, is a highly respected orthopedic surgeon in the United States who specializes in lower limb reconstructive surgery and trauma surgery. He knows as much as anyone in the world about hip and knee replacement surgery, in particular how to manage an infected or failed prosthesis. However, he would be the first to agree that being a skilled and well-trained specialist does not make someone an expert in overall health or preventing illness—not even the arthritic conditions that eventually require joint replacement.

It would be arrogant of physicians to feel that we are the only ones who have anything to say about health and wellness. There is a lot of wisdom in related health sciences and traditional healing practices that we need to be open to or at least aware of, as our patients are incorporating alternative practices in record numbers.

As is probably the case for many of us, my parents were my first role models for healthy living. My mother—a nurse—raised us on a healthy diet with fresh homemade meals since we were weaned, and my father grows enough fruits and vegetables for a small village in his large organic garden. Neither of my parents has stepped inside a fitness gym, yet both exercise vigorously every single day. At the time of this writing, they are both nearly ninety years old and still maintain a home in the city and a cottage at the lake, and lead full and vital lives. They are truly an inspiration and a blessing to me, and I will never tire of thanking them for the invaluable contributions they have made to the lives of their children and grandchildren.

It is also important to understand that many determinants of health and disease are controllable and therefore modifiable. While natural disasters, poverty and malnutrition are global problems with complex causes, nutrition is the single most important determinant of health that we can control. In developed countries, overeating and its disastrous, and escalating health fallout is now a larger problem than malnutrition. This is the first time in history that childhood obesity—because of excessive screen time and inactivity combined with supersized portions of junk food—has resulted in the projected life expectancy of this generation being lower than that of the parents' generation. The second greatest controllable risk factor is smoking and the third is hypertension (or elevated blood pressure).

Finally, I am concerned about the sustainability of the healthcare system in Canada, where I live and practise medicine. We are putting an increasing amount of resources into healthcare to the extent that over forty percent of our government spending goes towards diagnosing and treating illness. Despite these resources, we are not improving population health, empowering our citizens to make appropriate lifestyle choices, or protecting our environment for future generations. We are increasing our ability to treat disease without addressing the root causes of illness. A far greater emphasis needs to be placed on education, and this book is my small contribution to that cause. Beyond that, we need governments to create incentives for the population to become engaged in taking care of themselves and the world around us. Until that happens, all the money poured into healthcare is simply a band-aid on a wound that will never heal.

This book is organized into twelve habits. After reading the book, I suggest that you reread and reflect on one habit each month and, if your appetite is whetted, explore some of the reference books for that section. Think of *One Minute Medicine* as a kick-start to better health. If the book encourages you to re-evaluate your lifestyle in the interests of your own well-being, I will consider it a success.

To read about life changing stories from other readers of this book and to provide feedback go to:

www.oneminutemedicine.com

# REFERENCES

Of the many sources I consulted during the writing of *One Minute Medicine*, the following authors and works are ones I found most useful and interesting and often recommend to my patients.

## GENERAL

Weil, Dr. Andrew, 1983, Health and Healing, New York: Houghton Mifflin Co.
Dr. Andrew Weil (1942– ) is an American physician, best known for his work in the field of integrative medicine. He graduated from Harvard Medical School, and then studied ethnobotany—how people of a particular culture and region make use of indigenous plants, particularly for healing. The author of best-selling books, including *Spontaneous Healing; Eight Weeks to Optimum Health; Eating Well for Optimum Health, and Healthy Aging, and Spontaneous Happiness.* He also runs an informative website (www.drweil.com), where he answers questions relating to health. He is the founder and program director of the Arizona Center for Integrative Medicine, which he started in 1994 at the University of Arizona, Tucson, Arizona.

Robbins, John, 2001, *The Food Revolution, How Your Diet can help Save your Life and Our World*, Conari Press, Berkeley, California.

John Robbins (1947– ) is an American author who has explored the linkages between agriculture, health, and the environment. He graduated from the University of California,

Berkeley in 1969, and received a master's degree from Antioch College in 1976. Robbins advocates a plant-based diet for personal and environmental health. In 1987, he wrote *Diet for a New America*, an exposé on connections between diet, physical health, animal cruelty, and environmentalism. He updated these ideas in his 2001 book *The Food Revolution*, which includes information on organic food, genetically modified food, and factory farming. His 2006 book *Healthy at 100*, published by Random House, was printed on 100 percent post-consumer non-chlorine bleached paper, a first for a book from a major U.S. publisher. Check out www.johnrobbins.info for a wide selection of information related to health and the environment.

Chopra, Dr. Deepak, 1993, *Ageless Body, Timeless Mind—The Quantum Alternative to Growing Old.* Harmony Books.

Dr. Deepak Chopra (1946– ) is an endocrinologist, lecturer, and author of many books on spirituality and mind-body medicine. Born in New Delhi, India, he immigrated to the U.S. in 1968 with his wife, Rita. He practised Western medicine for many years but is also a proponent of Ayurveda—the traditional medicine of India. See his website: www.chopra.com

Dossey, Dr. Larry, 1993, *Healing Words: The Power of Prayer and the Practice of Medicine*, Harper Collins, 1999, *Reinventing Medicine—Beyond Mind-Body to a New Era of Healing*. Harper Collins, 2009, The Power of Premonitions: How Knowing the Future Can Shape Our Lives. Dutton, Published by Penguin Group, New York, USA.

Dr. Larry Dossey (1940 - ) is a distinguished Texas physician, who specialized in internal medicine. Through his research and writings he has become an internationally influential advocate of the role of the mind in health and the role of spirituality in healthcare. He is best known for his work on the healing power of prayer. See his website: www.dosseydossey.com

# REFERENCES BY TOPIC

## DIET

Weil, Dr. Andrew, 2000, *Eating Well for Optimum Health.* New York: Alfred A. Knopf.

Melina, Vesanto, Davis, Brenda and Harrison, Victoria, 1994, *Becoming Vegetarian.* Toronto: Macmillan Canada.

Béliveau, Richard and Gingras, Denis, 2005, Foods That Fight Cancer, and 2007, *Cooking with Foods That Fight Cancer,* Mc-Clelland and Stewart, Toronto, Canada.

Brand-Miller, Jennie, Wolever, Thomas, Colaguiri, Stephen, and Foster-Powell, Kaye, 1996, *Glucose Revolution, The Authoritative Guide to The Glycemic Index.* New York: Marlow & Company.

**www.glycemicindex.com** is the official website for the glycemic index which is based in the Human Nutrition Unit, School of Molecular and Microbial Biosciences, University of Sydney, Australia. The website is updated and maintained by the University's GI Group which includes research scientists and dieticians working in the area of glycemic index, health and nutrition including research into diet and weight loss, diabetes, and cardiovascular disease.

DASH diet (available on line and in print) is published by The National Institutes of Health, National Heart, Lung, and Blood Institute: A Guide to Lowering Your Blood Pressure with DASH.

Canada Food Guide—on the Heart and Stroke Foundation of Canada website: www.heartandstroke.com.

World Health Organization—The website: www.who.int contains useful information and guidelines regarding diet and population health.

## SMOKING CESSATION

Bryant, Dr. Simon, 1997, Know Smoking, *The Whole Truth about Smoking and Quitting*. Calgary: Middle Way Publishing Inc.

Ornish, Dr. Dean, 1990, *Dr. Dean Ornish's Program for Reversing Heart Disease*. New York: Ivy Books, Ballantine Books.

Practice guidelines for the treatment of patients with nicotine dependence. American Psychiatric Association, *American Journal of Psychiatry* Oct 1996; 153 (10 Supplement):1–31.

Raw, M., McNeill, A., West, R., Smoking cessation guidelines for health professionals: a guide to effective smoking cessation interventions for the health care system. *Thorax*, Dec 1998; 53 (Supplement 5 part 1):S1–S19.

Prochaska, James, Norcross, John and DiClemente, Carlo, 1994, *Changing For Good: the revolutionary program that explains the six stages of change and teaches you how to free yourself from bad habits.* New York: William Morrow and Company.

www.QuitNow.ca is a website sponsored by the government of British Columbia, Canada that offers counselling and other resources to help smokers quit.

http://www.ti.ubc.ca/pages/letter21.htm September-October, 1997, Effective Clinical Tobacco Intervention, Therapeutic Initiatives, University of British Columbia

**EXERCISE**

Cowley, Chris and Lodge, Dr. Henry. *Younger Next Year, Live Strong, Fit, and Sexy—Until You're 80 and Beyond.*, 2004, New York: Workman Publishing Co. Inc. Cowley and Lodge examine healthy aging and the important role of regular vigorous exercise in maintaining fitness and function into the eighties and beyond.

Karminoff, Leslie, 2007, Yoga Anatomy. Human Kinetics.

American Heart Association www.americanheart.org Physical Exercise in Daily Life.

## RELAXATION

Benson, Dr. Herbert, 1975, *The Relaxation Response*. New York: William Morrow and Co.

Weil, Dr. Andrew and Kabat-Zin, Dr. Jon, 2001, *Meditation for Optimum Health*, a two-CD program published by Sounds True, PO Box 8010 Boulder, CO, 80306.

Kabat-Zinn, Dr. Jon, 1991, *Full Catastrophe Living: Using the Wisdom of Your Body and Mind to Face Stress, Pain, and Illness*. Delta, and 1994, *Wherever You Go, There You Are: Mindfulness Meditation in Everyday Life*. Hyperion.

## SOCIAL CONNECTEDNESS

Putnam, Robert D., 2000, Bowling Alone, *The Collapse and Revival of American Community*. Simon & Shuster.

Bentall, David C, 2004, *The Company You Keep: The Transforming Power of Male Friendship*. Augsberg Books, Minneapolis.

Wexler, Mark, 2003, *The Four Faces of Capitalism: Structure and Change in Organizations*, Vancouver: Simon Fraser University, Harbour Centre Campus, prepublication copy.

## SLEEP

Coren, Stanley, 1996, *Sleep Thieves, An Eye-opening Exploration into the Science and Mysteries of Sleep*. New York: The Free Press.

Hauri, Peter and Linde, Shirley, 1996, *No More Sleepless Nights.* Barnes & Noble.

CBTforInsomnia.com is a program developed by Dr. Gregg Jacobs at Harvard Medical School. Cognitive-behavioral therapy (CBT) is the only scientifically proven non-drug insomnia treatment. Unlike most sleep help programs, CBT teaches you how to stop insomnia. CBT is a natural remedy that has no side effects.

**SPIRITUALITY**

*The Holy Bible* ("New American Bible"): any print or on-line edition.

Borg, Marcus. ed., 2002, *The Parallel Sayings of Jesus and the Buddha*. Duncan Baird Publishers. This work outlines the striking similarity in the message of the New Testament and that of ancient Buddhist scriptures.

Kelly, Matthew, 2010, *Rediscovering Catholicism, A Spiritual Guide to Living with Passion and Purpose*, Beacon Publishing.

**CHANGE MANAGEMENT**

Amen, Daniel, *Change Your Brain, Change Your Life, The Breakthrough Program for Conquering Anxiety, Depression, Obsessiveness, Anger, and Impulsiveness*, 1999, Three Rivers Press, New York, discusses Cognitive Behavioural Therapy—change how you think to improve mood and health, *Change Your Brain Change Your Body: Use Your Brain to Get and Keep the Body You*

*Have Always Wanted*, 2010, Three Rivers Press, New York

Kotter, John. The website www.kotterinternation.com and the 8 Step Change Model describe the principles of organizational change management as described by Harvard Business School professor John Kotter. His 8 Step Change Model can also be applied to personal change.

Fisher, John. For a discussion on the reaction to change, refer to John Fisher's stages of personal transition in the process of change: http://www.businessballs.com/personalchangeprocess.htm

Abreshoff, Captain D. Michael, 2002, *It's Your Ship. Management Techniques from the Best Damn Ship in the Navy.* New York; Warner Books.

**AGING**

Weil, Dr. Andrew, 2005, *Healthy Aging, A Lifelong Guide to Your Physical and Spiritual Well-Being.* New York: Alfred A. Knopf

Cowley, Chris, and Dr. Henry Lodge, 2004, *Younger Next Year, Live Strong, Fit, and Sexy Until You're 80 and Beyond.* New York: Workman Publishing.

Snowdon, David, 2001, *Aging With Grace, What the Nun Study Teaches Us About Leading Longer Healthier and More Meaningful Lives.* Bantam, 2001

Vaillant, George, 2002, *Aging Well: Surprising Guideposts to a Happier Life from the Landmark Harvard Study of Adult*

*Development*. Little, Brown and Company, Boston.

**PURPOSE AND BALANCE**

Phillips, Dave, 2006, *Three Big Questions—everyone asks sooner or later,* www.dphillips.com.

Weil, Dr Andrew, 1997, *8 Weeks to Optimum Health*, Alfred Knopf, New York.

Chopra, Dr. Deepak, 1991, *Perfect Health—The Complete Mind Body Guide*, Three Rivers Press, New York.

Wooden, John and Carty, Jay, 2005, *Pyramid of Success: Building Blocks for a Better Life*, Regal Books, Ventura, California.

Posen, Dr. David B. *Always Change a Losing Game and Work-Life Balance* 1994, Print and Tape editions. www.davidposen.com

Suzuki, David with Amanda McConnell, 1997, *The Sacred Balance—Rediscovering our Place in Nature*, David Suzuki Foundation, Greystone Books, Douglas & McIntyre Publishing Group, The Mountaineers, Vancouver/Toronto

Murphy, Jim, 2010, *Inner Excellence—Achieve Extraordinary Business Success Through Mental Toughness.* New York: McGraw-Hill. Jim Murphy is a performance coach who works with elite athletes, teams, and corporations. He helps them to find balance and fulfillment on the field, at the office and in the home through a success model based on love, wisdom, and courage. Find him at innerexcellence.com.

# INDEX

# PRAISE FOR ONE MINUTE MEDICINE *continued*

"Dr. Spangehl's ONE MINUTE MEDICINE is not only a handbook to vibrant health but a common-sense guide to happier living. The simple remedies he suggests are easy to fit into even the most hectic of schedules. His realistic narrative of an individual re-claiming his lost health is a compelling read and gently steers us towards a brighter, healthier future."
— **Russ Hiebert**, BA, MBA, LL.B., Member of Parliament

"I love this book! ONE MINUTE MEDICINE, through clear and engaging storytelling, provides a precious gift – how to reframe our lives as we strive to reach our full potential! In this complex world, this book provides a cornerstone to build our lives on – it will be a game changer!!"
— **Kathy Kinloch**, President, Vancouver Community College

"A medical book that's a "page turner"? Who would have thought it possible? But Werner has pulled it off. ONE MINUTE MEDICINE is interesting and engaging, yet concise and thorough. Read it every evening for a week. It's the perfect prescription for what ails you."
— **Jay Carty**, Former L.A. Laker, speaker, and author of twelve books including best sellers *COACH WOODEN ONE-ON-ONE* and *COACH WOODEN'S PYRAMID OF SUCCESS*